PEOPLE WITH MS

WITH THE

COURAGE TO GIVE

PEOPLE WITH MS
WITH THE
Courage to Give

JACKIE WALDMAN

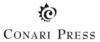

CONARI PRESS

First published in 2003 by Conari Press,
an imprint of Red Wheel/Weiser, LLC
York Beach, ME
With offices at:
368 Congress Street
Boston, MA 02210
www.redwheelweiser.com

Library of Congress Cataloging-in-Publication Data

Waldman, Jackie.
  People with MS with the courage to give / Jackie Waldman.
    p. cm.
  ISBN 1-57324-923-8
  1. Multiple sclerosis--Patients--Biography. I. Title.
  RC377.W355 2003
  362.1'96834'00922--dc21   2003009979

Typeset in ITC Berkeley Oldstyle

Printed in Canada
Transcontinental Press

10   09   08   07   06   05   04   03
8   7   6   5   4   3   2   1

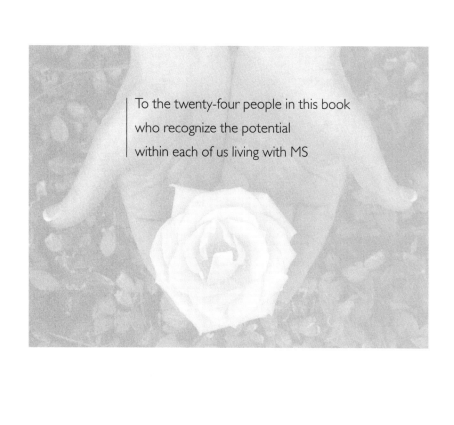

To the twenty-four people in this book
who recognize the potential
within each of us living with MS

CONTENTS

The support I received for this book was overwhelmingly generous. I am grateful.

My heartfelt thanks go to all of my friends at Biogen for making this book possible and for supporting my efforts to raise awareness about MS.

Thanks to Arney Rosenblat at the National Multiple Sclerosis Society and others in Society chapters across the country for helping me locate possible contributors. Their recommendations proved to be exactly right for this book.

Special thanks go to the friends at Spectrum Science Public Relations, Berlex, Serono, Teva, Fleishman-Hillard, Inc., and Betaseron Champions of Courage for putting me in touch with some of the courageous people whose stories are shared in the book.

Thanks to all of the wonderful staff at Red Wheel/Weiser/Conari. I am blessed to be associated with a publisher who has expertise and a passion for helping others. Jan and Michael, I am grateful. Special thanks to Caroline Pincus for expert editing and Brenda Knight, Kathleen Fivel, Jill Rogers, Lucine Kasbarian, and Chris Wold for all their help in making this book.

When an author has the same publicist for four years, there's a very good reason—she's good. Thanks to Karen Frost, publicist extraordinaire and dear friend for believing in the courage to give message and her persistence with the media.

Who would imagine a New York literary agent excited for an author who decides to donate all of her royalties to the National MS Society? My thanks go to my kind agent and friend, Jim Levine.

I thank my family, Steve, Melissa and Bart, Todd, and Michael for their love and encouragement, for their laughter, and for what we learn together every day.

Thank you.
—Jackie

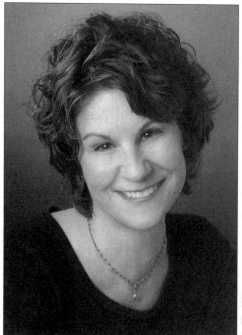

John Tilley, 2002

I SEEMED TO BE LEADING A CHARMED LIFE.

At age fourteen I had a date with a handsome guy named Steve. He took me to a Dallas Chaparrals basketball game and then to the lake where all the couples went. He took a blanket and a guitar out of the trunk of his car. And as we sat at the edge of the still water under a moonlit sky, that fifteen-year-old boy sang the most beautiful songs in the world to me, revealing his gentle soul. I knew at that moment that I had met my soulmate.

Steve and I married and lived in Dallas, where he joined his family's business and I taught children with special needs, but later resigned to stay at home with our three children, Melissa, Todd, and Michael. My life was filled with soccer games, gymnastic carpools, school carpools, school plays, friends, family gatherings, and the athletics that were always so important to me. I went to aerobics class every day, sometimes twice a day, and jogged three to five miles a day.

As our children got older, I started my own business. I got the idea from a girl I met on the beach while I was in Hawaii with Steve on a business trip. She was making hair bows and taught me how to make a simple bow, too. For the rest of the vacation, she and I spent every morning on the beach in Maui making bows while our husbands were in meetings.

I bought ribbon and wire and made bows during the long flight home. When an airline attendant asked if she could buy some bows for her daughter, I told her, "No way. Here, take these." She explained it was against airline regulation to accept free gifts, so we agreed on $5 per bow. My hair accessory business, Bow Jangles, was born.

And it grew. My competitive nature, which drove my love for athletics, drove me in business too. Before long, I had twenty-five employees and twenty-five sales reps across the country. We were in every major department store and hundreds of small boutiques. During the Gulf War, we made and sold thousands of red, white, and blue bows.

When I first started my business, it was fun and more fun. But, as it grew and became more successful, it also became more stressful. Before I knew it, I was getting to the office at 6:30 AM every morning and scrambling to run it without sacrificing quality family life.

It was around that time that I started having a strange tingling sensation around my waist. At first I thought I was just imagining it. Then I attributed it to stress. But when the tingling progressed down my legs to my toes, and my legs became numb, I went to the doctor. After examining me, he told me to see a neurologist immediately.

The neurologist, a friend of ours, hospitalized me that day. I had MRIs of my upper and lower spine and brain. The next day, they did a spinal tap. I'll never forget lying on my stomach, with a needle in my spine, hearing one nurse whisper to another, "What are they testing for?"

The other nurse answered, "multiple sclerosis."

I lifted my head and asked, "Is that what 'Jerry's Kids' have?"

The nurses were embarrassed that I had overheard them and quickly reassured me it wasn't. But, at that point I knew this was serious.

On July 12, 1991—I'll never forget that day—the doctor walked into my room and told me and Steve that I had multiple sclerosis. Even the doctor seemed sad.

The doctor went on to tell us that multiple sclerosis—MS—is an autoimmune disease, meaning that the body attacks itself. He explained that nerves have a coating around them made of myelin, kind of the way telephone wires are wrapped in insulation. When the telephone insulation is torn, the message we hear in the phone sounds garbled. Similarly, when myelin is torn or destroyed, messages can't flow smoothly along the nerves. And that's what my problem was. The MRI of my brain showed scars where the myelin had been destroyed. That's why my legs weren't functioning. He suggested several doctors who specialized in MS.

Steve and I held each other and cried. We were so frightened. Through my tears, I told him how sorry I was. Through his tears, he told me to quit apologizing. He told me we'd get through this together.

We chose a doctor, and he came to visit that same day. I will always remember his kind and gentle manner. After reassuring me I wasn't going to die, he told me that even though my legs were numb then, that didn't mean they would be numb forever. He told us of the different types of MS and he suspected mine to be relapsing-remitting.

As the doctor explained it, our first priority was to halt this attack. We tried IV steroids first, but that didn't help. Then we tried chemotherapy. With that, some feeling returned to my legs. I was so excited, so hopeful. The doctor allowed me to go home and have the next two rounds of chemo at home with visiting nurses.

At home, I had to face our children, who were in middle school and high school at the time. Steve was right there with me. We told each of them that I would not die from this and that MS is not hereditary. I then promised them that nothing would change.

But, of course, everything did change.

After I finished chemo and got my strength back, I assumed I would be fine. I tried to ignore the overwhelming fatigue I felt on a daily basis. I pushed myself forward, believing that if I just tried hard enough, I would beat this disease—even though I had read there was no known cure.

One day when Steve and the children were gone, I got on the treadmill and fast-walked three miles. Sweat poured out of me triumphantly. I was so excited to be able to exercise so well again. I told myself I was feeling normal. Everything would be fine. But after I cooled down, I had to sleep for four hours.

Looking back, I realize I was in complete denial—big time denial.

When I finally quit denying that I had a serious illness, I became very angry. Why me? Why was God punishing me? What had I done so wrong? Did I get this disease as a payback for the fact that my life had gone so well? That things had come easily for me? How fair is this?

I asked these angry questions over and over and over. They went through my mind continuously. I wasn't really looking for any answers. I was just asking out of anger.

Because I wasn't able to work full-time anymore, I had to close my business and sell the entire inventory. I had acquired a partner. You can imagine how badly I felt disappointing her, Steve, and myself.

I had ruined an absolutely perfect life.

Terrible thoughts began to run through my mind. Would Steve be better off without me, with a vibrant wife who could still dance and go out spontaneously? Maybe I should just pack my bags and leave. What if my family is just pretending to still love me? When they are alone with their thoughts, do they really resent me?

Throughout everything—and no matter what I was feeling inside—I outwardly maintained a positive, cheery appearance. I made sure MS was not the focus in our home. The kids' schoolwork, outside interests, and social calendars never suffered. When friends called, I said I was "fine." When family called, I was "fine." If people offered help, I said I didn't need it.

I was even "fine" for Steve. I knew he felt my pain and devastation. But I couldn't bring myself to talk openly about my feelings with him. I didn't want to feel his pain. I just couldn't face it. I had enough of my own.

I did have one dear friend, Dee, whom I could unload to. She understood me almost better than I understood myself. She had two rocking chairs on her front porch, and we spent many, many hours just rocking and talking. I often thought how good it was those chairs couldn't talk—they knew way too much.

Many days Dee made me angry with her peaceful, forgiving manner. I was frustrated by her daily affirmations, her quest for inner peace. I told her the philosophy she lived was easy for her to embrace—but just wait until she suffered in some way. And that's when she told me about her childhood, about growing up with an alcoholic single mom, about being on her own by the time she was seventeen, about having faith and choosing love.

I'd leave her house thinking about how impressed I was with her courage. It didn't occur to me to think about how I could apply her philosophy to my life with MS.

When the movie *Schindler's List* was released, Dee and I went to see it. After the movie, we talked about the power of Oskar Schindler's courage and kindness—saving over one thousand lives and, indirectly, all the future generations that would be born to those people. We talked about the courage of the people during the Holocaust.

We began to brainstorm the idea of a week in Dallas celebrating the value of kindness as part of the National Random Acts of Kindness™ Month. And we decided to turn our ideas into reality.

The week of February 7–14, 1995, changed my life. Rosa Parks, Martin Luther King III, W. Deen Mohammed, and Dennis Weaver came to Dallas and spoke at kindness rallies, at schools, and at interfaith services. We had a kindness rally for 10,000 school children. Some of the acts of kindness Dallas experienced were the girls from the YWCA handing out hot chocolate to downtown workers as they left their buildings, children's art exhibits depicting kindness, interfaith services, children and adult choirs singing in the malls, and even the Dallas police handing out kindness citations.

For the very first time since my MS diagnosis, I was giving to others and not thinking about myself. My motivation for the week had been my admiration for the courageous Holocaust survivors, for making kindness more powerful than violence. I felt better than I had felt since being diagnosed.

I realized true survival isn't about my legs working or overcoming fatigue; true survival is survival of our spirit, no matter what. After seeing *Schindler's List* and Kindness Week my pity party ended.

I then trained to become a docent at the Dallas Memorial Center for Holocaust Studies. Soon I was speaking with fifty middle school students each week, taking them on tours of the center. During each tour, I would become emotional when I told them about one particular survivor. He was their age—fourteen years old—when he was taken to the camps. He lost his parents, brothers, and sisters. You'd expect him to be angry. He was one of the kindest, most courageous persons I've had the honor to know; he was the founder of this memorial center. He took his loss and pain and used it as an opportunity. He wanted students and adults to learn about the Holocaust so it could never happen again.

When I heard about a group of girls in Dallas who can't live in their own homes because it isn't safe, I knew I wanted to work with them. One Thanksgiving, the girls, my sister-in-law, and I prepared a feast complete with decorations. We sat around the table, held hands, and each girl expressed what made her feel grateful. I heard these girls who can't even live at home express their gratitude for friendship, love, and comfortable shelter. They continued to teach me courage when they surprised me and showed up for the MS Walk that spring with pledges and the desire to help find a cure for MS.

A pattern in my life began to become clear. As I was working with those who had suffered and felt their courage, I was learning how to find the courage to live with MS, how to find the courage to give.

As with the Holocaust survivor and the girls at Our Friends' Place, by putting aside pain—physical and mental—long enough to reach out and give to others, I was seeing how to begin to heal. There may be no cure for MS, but there is a cure for the anger, sadness, and fear, and the very people I was giving to were teaching me how to find my courage. I finally understood that my MS is a part of who I am, but only a very small part.

Shortly afterward, I had a very powerful dream. A book was laid out for me. I was to find thirty people who had suffered physical and/or emotional pain and gone beyond it to help someone else. I needed to interview them and share their stories in their own voices.

I woke up knowing I had to live this dream. My first book, *The Courage to Give,* published by Conari Press, tells thirty stories of people who have had something happen to them physically and/or emotionally, yet when they started helping others their lives changed miraculously—just as I dreamed it to be.

When a producer from the *Oprah* show called me the day after *The Courage to Give* was released, I was sure it was a friend playing a joke. But it was no joke; I had been invited on the show. Within thirty-six hours of the show's airing, more than 7,500 people had signed up to volunteer with a charity they had found on the Website I suggested during the show—*www.volunteermatch.org.*

Since then, I have compiled four more books of inspiring stories about people who have overcome adversity in their lives by finding the courage to give: *Teens with the Courage to Give; America, September 11: The Courage to Give* (a fundraiser raising $28,000 to date for the New York Firefighter's Fund), *Teachers with the Courage to Give,* and now this book, *People with MS with the Courage to Give,* a fundraiser for the National MS Society (see page 164 for more information about the Society).

You'll read about Anthony Zaremba, whose days spent gardening filled his soul. He used to paint, and after losing use of his right hand he had to teach himself to paint with his left hand. After three years, he could successfully paint again. He is in a wheelchair, so since he can't garden anymore, he would listen to classical music and paint as his wife gardened. He won a grant to build accessible community garden plots not only for individuals with MS, but for all people with disabilities.

You'll meet Sister Karen who will tell you, "Whenever I begin to feel alone, I try to remember to reach out to a friend to help me do errands, pray with me, or just talk. Prayer is probably the most healing thing I do. In the morning, I pour myself a cup of coffee, light a candle, and pray the psalms. I am always struck by the ones that speak of healing. From praying the psalms, my thinking changes from what I *can't* do with MS to what I *can*."

You'll meet Jean Griswold who tells us, "For thirty-seven years I've struggled with the increasingly frustrating ravages of this disease. For the last ten years I have been unable to walk or to even stand. I can't even get from my bed to my wheelchair without a Hoyer lift. Yet I still go to work every day because I have a dream and am still living it. My work of providing care to the homebound has helped 60,000 people. What could be better than that?"

You'll meet Pam Allen, whose love of and talent for playing softball was taken away due to MS. She mourned her loss until she was asked to fill in as coach for her daughter's soccer team and, amazingly, began to realize that that was "one of the best things that could've happened to me. For the first time in over a year I was not focused on myself and the disease. I found myself looking forward to practice, and I just loved teaching the kids the sport that I had loved for so many years! I learned so much that summer and felt like I had been given a fresh start at a new life! I learned that if I focused on helping others, and not on myself and the disease, my life could still be as fun and exciting as it had been before MS. That was a life-changing revelation."

Meeting twenty-four new friends, people who have endured the ravages of MS yet are reaching out in their own way to give to others, reminds me daily of the miracles of life. For those of you with MS who, like me, have had difficulty getting past the challenges of our disease, the contributors you're about to meet will give you hope. Each is living their passion, doing what they love, despite numbness, poor eyesight, inability to walk, overwhelming fatigue, poor balance, other symptoms, and altered lifestyles. Yes, that takes courage. But, because they have discovered their unique gifts to share, their lives have become rich and fulfilling—much larger than living with MS.

Recently I found a newspaper clipping featuring me as a child with two other children. It was in the *Dallas Times Herald,* in 1956. I was four years old. The caption reads, "Socks Away—three tiny members of Temple Emanu-El sort through 563 pairs of socks they and fellow church school members have collected for the City-County Department of Public Welfare to give needy youngsters at Christmas. The children gave socks to the program in place of exchanging gifts among themselves."

I cried looking at the joy and love in my little face. At four years old, I had known the peace and joy of service to others. But, for so many years, I had forgotten the truth of that little girl. I cried tears of gratitude for the gift of remembering who I really am.

I cried for the miracle of life, for the chance I and we all have been given to offer our unique gifts to the world, gifts born, so often, from our very woundedness.

So now I invite you to meet my new friends. These are wonderful people— all of whom continue to inspire, motivate, and teach me a lesson I had once known long ago but had forgotten. These people have the courage we all need, the courage to see beyond our MS. The admiration and love I feel in my heart for each of them will stay with me always. Their stories have changed me, as I hope they will change you.

I thank each of them for revealing their stories to us.

CHAPTER 1

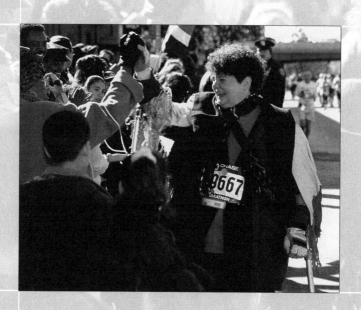

No Lifetime Guarantees

ZOE KOPLOWITZ

LIFE AT ITS LONGEST is way too short. We don't get to choose whether or not we have MS, but from moment to moment we do get to choose how to live with it. If we spend every waking moment either waiting for "The Cure" or waiting for the other shoe to drop, then we don't just *have* a disease, we *are* one. The difference between these two states is far more than just a matter of semantics. It's about the quality of life. _____

When I was initially diagnosed with MS thirty years ago, I was really angry. Because I was so young—only twenty-five at the time—I believed that God owed me a guarantee on the body and all of its parts. I really believed that God had come down personally and done this to me.

Back in those days there were no ABCR drugs, there was nothing. A diagnosis of MS was virtually a death sentence. They gave you a pat on the head, told you to go home and hope for the best, and, if you were religious, to pray.

I walked around angry for several months, really ticked off. Then one day I was riding the bus home from work and a much older man, in his late eighties, fell down at my feet and died of a massive heart attack holding onto my hand.

The only thing that I ever knew about him was that his name was Joseph, but in his ending was a new beginning for me. I realized then and there that God and the world didn't owe me anything. Not one single thing. There are no guarantees in life. Not for anyone. You get what you get in life and what you do with it is totally up to you. As for the answer to that most unanswerable of questions "Why me?" perhaps the answer was far simpler than I had suspected. Maybe the answer could be summed up in six letters. Two very simple words: "Why not?" Pithy. Succinct. And Zen. Very Zen.

I decided that whether I had a week or a day, I needed to make the best of it, the most of it.

If I had to accept this unpredictable intruder known as MS as my lifetime companion, then let it take on meaning and function in my life. Let it serve as my teacher. Let me learn from it whatever life lessons I'm meant to learn. Let me become the ever-vigilant student so that some day I may become the teacher. Let this be the purpose of my soul.

A couple of weeks after the incident on the bus I was walking by an appliance store that had a whole bunch of television sets in the window. Only one of them was plugged in and turned on. On that TV set was nothing but static, and as I watched it, I couldn't move. It dawned on me that that was how I'd been leading my life since my diagnosis. I'd been acting as if I was trapped in front of a TV set with static on it. That's when I formulated my "TV set theory of life." I really believe that when we're born God and the world gives every single one of us a TV set with hundreds of channels. Endless opportunities to learn and to grow. One channel has static. My static channel happens to have MS on it. Everybody in the world has their own static channel. I realized that I could sit in front of that static channel for the rest of my life or I could get up and change the channel. I decided to do the latter.

That doesn't mean I never have a bad day, but it does mean that I limit my pity parties to a half hour. I know for a fact that every minute I spend feeling sorry for myself is a minute I'll never get back.

Over the years, I believe, I really have changed the channels on my personal TV. I've had good times, good jobs, and good friends. Sure, living with an unpredictable disease makes some things more difficult, but in the end, they are all doable.

Well, that philosophy worked pretty well for more than fifteen years. Then, in January 1988, I developed a terrible case of bronchitis. Since I'm a believer in trying natural things first, I was taking a huge dose of vitamin C. Not the time-released gel caps of the twenty-first century, but those big old horse pills. One of the pills lodged in my throat and I literally started to choke to death—on a vitamin C tablet! A friend of mine was there and he did the Heimlich maneuver. He started CPR and saved my life. Up to that point I had believed that I would certainly perish from something related to MS. Realizing that I could choke to death on a vitamin pill, that such things happen, was another huge wake-up call for me.

Since being diagnosed with MS I had more or less given up on the physical parts of life. I had focused most of my attention on the cerebral, the emotional, and the spiritual. But the vitamin pill incident made me realize that I wanted back everything I had surrendered to MS. I wanted it more than I had ever wanted anything in my life. I decided I had to make something amazing happen in order to celebrate what I saw as the second half of my life. It had to be something so outrageous that it would take everything that I had and still more—something that would help me reinvent myself and reclaim my physicality. That was when I decided to run my first New York City Marathon.

I had absolutely no idea how to run a marathon; I just knew that I would. I pictured myself crossing the finish line wearing a designer tracksuit, wind blowing in my hair. Of course that was not the real picture at all.

Then I decided that I was going to do it without appliances. Back then I could still get by some days without a cane. But I couldn't take more than eight or ten steps before falling on my face, so I went out and bought some hockey pads for my knees and my elbows and a crash helmet. Another unrealistic picture of how I would cross the finish line. Then I realized that I could have either my little fantasy of crossing the finish line or I could have the real thing, and if I wanted the real thing, I had to find out how to get it.

I called Road Runners, the governing body of the New York City Marathon, and they put me in touch with an organization called the Achilles Track Club—an international running club for disabled athletes. Thanks to them, I began my real training.

When I first decided to do the marathon, I made a list of all my assets and the reasons I believed I could do it: a highly developed sense of the absurd, a really great sense of humor, the ability to achieve long-term goals that require planning and multitasking. These were at the top of my list.

Then I made a list of all my deficits, potential liabilities that might thwart my plans or put a damper on my dreams: limited eye-hand coordination, unsteady gait, no strength or endurance.

And finally, I made a third list—of all the ways I could fix the items on the second list. I tend to think up very tactile, down-to-earth strategies. I realized I could play pinball to improve my eye-hand coordination; I could enroll in an Afro-Brazilian dance class to improve my gait; I could do weight training to improve my stamina and endurance.

For almost ten months that first year I trained with an amazing support team. In the beginning I could only do five blocks one way and five blocks back, but that's exactly the trick. Just as you do with anything in life, you build and you build and you build.

In November 1988 I "ran" my first marathon in nineteen hours and fifty-seven minutes. It was the fastest race I have ever run. Over the years, my times have ranged from nineteen to thirty-three hours. To date, I have completed a total of seventeen marathons, fifteen in New York, one in Boston, and one in London.

As I've gotten older, of course, I've gotten slower. Also, I'm now a diabetic, so every two miles I have to stop and check my blood sugar and look at my feet for blisters because I have neuropathy so bad I wouldn't know it if I got a blister.

Folks are always amazed that I'm able to do 26.2 miles and stay awake for more than twenty-four hours. The truth is that there are no magic tricks. No smoke and mirrors. Like any major goal, I just break it down into a series of manageable stages. The first year it was a mystery, an unknown adventure. Now I plan things differently. I know that a certain person will be there to support me at mile three, that there will be a coffee break at mile five and a bathroom break at mile seven. Just like everything else, if we look at it as one long never-ending road, it's completely overwhelming, but if we break it down into smaller segments with treats interspersed, then the miles become doable fragments, proving once again that the whole really is greater than the sum of its parts.

People often ask me which of my marathons was the most memorable. Hands down. No contest. November 2001.

On September 11, 2001, I was working three blocks from the World Trade Center as a third shift supervisor for an employment agency. The only reason I was spared was that my first shift replacement was five minutes late. If she had been on time, I would have been standing at the bus stop under the twin towers when the first plane hit. The woman who was standing there was doused with seventy gallons of jet fuel oil. She died six weeks later. Along with tens of thousands of New Yorkers I barely escaped with my life that day.

For a long time, I grappled with the memory of everything I had seen and heard on that terrible day. Why did I get to live when so many others perished?

Someone was five minutes late and I'm still here. If she had been on time I surely would have perished. Was life really this random or was there a divine plan to things? After thinking about it and praying over it for a long time I realized it really didn't matter which was true. The point really was that *I am still here,* and I know without a doubt that each day that I live is bonus time. Another day for me to rededicate myself to my missions in life—dedicating myself to the fight against MS and traveling around the country helping people reinvent the words *win* and *achieve.*

I completed the 2001 New York City Marathon in a little over twenty-eight hours. What an extraordinary day. Thirty thousand runners took back our city one block at a time. For many of us it was the beginning of the healing process that continues to this day.

Ultimately, for me, a marathon is far more than a big race cut into bite-sized pieces. It's a metaphor for life. It's about doing that thing that we think we can't do. It's about moving past where we would ordinarily give up in real life and knowing that once we have done so, no one can ever tell us we can't do something we really want to do. We know both literally and metaphorically that we have what it takes to go the distance in life.

I really believe that 99 percent of the people in this country do marathons every single day of their lives in one way or another. They raise children, work second jobs, live with MS, and so on. All those things are marathons. A marathon is not just a "run" in terms of miles, but is about the intensity and commitment with which we lead our lives. For all we are and all we do, we need to give ourselves the finishers' medals we deserve.

Over the years the MS, diabetes, and the marathon have certainly been excellent teachers. They've taught me the value of humor, faith, and discipline. They've shown me that humility and vulnerability are the precursors to strength. I know

now that winning is not always and necessarily about being first. It can be, but it doesn't have to be.

No, winning is about doing everything you do from the center of your being, with everything you've got. Winning is about having a dream and implementing a plan. It's about viewing those unforeseen, adverse circumstances that appear to block our way as lessons and opportunities. Ultimately winning is about putting one foot in front of the other until we get where we have to go in life. No doubt about it, in any life there's a lot of hard work to be done. But along the way there's so much magic to be had.

I have a poster taped to my bedroom wall. It's the last thing I see before falling asleep and the first thing I see on rising. It is a picture of a nameless, faceless runner on what appears to be an endless road, with the caption, "The race belongs not only to the swift and the strong, but to those who keep on running."

Words to live by.

Editor's note: For many years Zoe led a team of runners called the Marathon Strides Against MS. The team raised more than $2 million for research and programs.

To learn more of Zoe's story, see her book *The Winning Spirit: Life Lessons Learned in Last Place,* Doubleday, 1997.

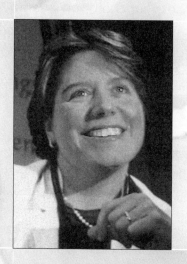

CHAPTER 2

When Doctor Became Patient

DR. ALICIA CONILL

T HOSE OF US CHOSEN, in a seemingly random way, by chronic illness also have a choice to make—the choice to live. I made that choice on a damp November day in 1995. Each morning that I struggle from bed to my wheelchair, or each night that leg spasms and pain keep me awake, I choose again. ———————————————————

It should have come as no surprise. Everyone I have ever spoken to about MS, as a physician or as a fellow patient, tells me there are always warning signs. Episodes of discomfort that pass. The activities you start avoiding without realizing it out of fear of triggering those "silly" symptoms. For me, it was an intense dislike of hot weather, occasional blurring of vision, and transient numbness and tingling. Well, certainly the fatigue could be explained. I was training to be a doctor and sleep was a luxury—and not one I indulged in often enough. I had reason to be tired.

I figured I would join an academic clinical practice where I would care for patients and teach students and residents the science, and even more importantly, the art of medicine. My schedule would finally allow for sleep. Even after my dear grandmother was diagnosed with an expanding abdominal aortic aneurysm and needed surgery, from which she developed complications that would result in an almost six-month ICU stay, I continued to believe that modern medicine would prevail in restoring her to good health and I would check in with a daily phone call and occasional weekend visit. Wrong.

Every night I would board a train from Philadelphia to NYC, catnap in a chair next to my grandmother's bed, and board the 6 A.M. train back to Philly. Then, I began inpatient rounds and outpatient office hours. Admittedly, I held the innocent notion all young doctors share. I thought I was invincible. Wrong again.

After six months, my grandmother died, but not before the first sign surfaced that something was really wrong with me. I had already developed transient blindness in my right eye, which lasted approximately eight weeks before resolving spontaneously, and a persistent numbing and squeezing sensation from my butt and crotch area to my toes. But I convinced myself that the transient blindness was a corneal abrasion and the diffuse numbness a slipped disc.

Looking back, I am of course embarrassed at this admission. I believe I am an excellent diagnostician, but everything changes when doctor becomes patient. Fear and denial overcame all my diagnostic skills. Did I know? Yes, I knew. But, I wasn't going to be the one to break the news to myself. When the wise and kind neurologist said, "This is multiple sclerosis," some part of me wasn't really surprised.

Nine years later, on a crisp fall day, the colors around me vibrant and breathtaking, I accepted a friend's invitation to a barbecue even though I would only know a handful of people there. Of course people asked. "Alicia, what do you do?" I paused and replied, "I *used to be* a doctor." My friend looked at me in dismay and interjected, "You're still are a doctor!" What my friend didn't know is that only a week earlier, in a voice lacking emotion, eyes avoiding mine, my neurologist (obviously not the same one who confirmed my diagnosis) told me that I was now totally disabled and could no longer practice my profession.

It was just a routine visit. I expressed my concern about loss of sensation on the tip of each finger, which sometimes interfered with my ability to confidently perform physical examinations. I had to take extra time to be sure I did not miss a bump, a lump, or alterations in the rhythm and intensity of pulses. I had already cut back on office hours because the symptoms were always worse after long days, and at this point I had been using a three-wheel scooter for several years. Most of my patients were aware of my diagnosis, especially as it affected my legs. This new symptom, however, was invisible to the naked eye and easier to hide from others and deny to myself.

But there was no denial or hiding this time. I took an oath to *primum non nocere* (first, do no harm) and had always taken that oath very seriously in caring for people who entrusted their lives to me. So, I shared the symptoms with my physician, knowing full well that this would change my life for some time, possibly forever.

Silly me, I thought the neurologist might acknowledge the major loss this represented. No such luck. I received neither healing nor curing nor caring from him during that visit. He just said I should send him any papers I might need to fill out for permanent disability.

Leaving his office, the physical numbness in my legs seemed to spread and surround my entire being. If I could not be a doctor in the way I had been, if I had to close my practice and let go of a patient panel of over three thousand, if I had to hang up my white coat and stethoscope, who was I? The downward spiral had begun.

For a painfully long time, I had no answer. My sense of self was so closely tied to being a physician that I feared I would be nothing, be worth nothing, without it. I had always wanted to heal people. My mother still has my kindergarten report card that says, "Alicia wants to be a doctor." When I was seven, my parents gave me a nurse's outfit for Christmas; I was infuriated and said, "I don't want to be a nurse—I want to be a doctor."

Many times I had prescribed counseling and medication for patients with clinical depression. I had given numerous talks about how to recognize and treat it. The warning signs were ingrained in my memory as if etched in stone. But I was a patient now and could not even access my own best advice. The descent continued. Accelerating it was the fact that my personal life had started to unravel as well. Truth be told, I came dangerously close to ending my life, but forces came together at just the right time, in just the right way, and led me out of my descent. I chose to live. Only then did I envision the difference I could still make. I would share the lessons learned through my experience as physician and patient.

I had become concerned about doctor burnout and loss of empathy. Empathy has been defined as "your pain in my heart." It reflects understanding, but means more than understanding in a rational or mental way. It requires an ability to feel, care, and connect on an emotional level. Empathy is a critical component of healing. But it is not exactly emphasized in medical school. In fact, medical residents may find empathy reservoirs dangerously low after the stress and demands of residency. And these are the very people on the frontline of caring for the chronically ill, the disabled, the critically ill, and the dying.

The fact is, most residents are young and have not had any personal experience of illness or physical impairment. They have only viewed illness from the outside looking in. What happens to these young, idealistic men and women? What happens after they take their oath on graduation day and promise to first do no harm? Does our medical education provide any specific interventions during postgraduate training to foster a continued sense of medicine as an art, of communication as a critical diagnostic and therapeutic tool? Can empathy be taught? Those were just a few of the questions I started asking.

In 1998, in an attempt to search for answers, I founded the Conill Institute for Chronic Illness. Its inaugural project was a program called the Disability Experience,© which would be an experiential seminar lasting up to twenty-six hours. The principle behind experiential learning is that by actually having the experience (even in a controlled setting), the learner will appreciate what it is like to "walk in their shoes" or "to sit in their wheelchair."

For the Disability Experience,© future doctors and caregivers would be put into wheelchairs for extended periods and assigned simple tasks like getting out of bed or going to the store. Bottle caps would be put in their mouths so they would know what it's like to try to speak after a stroke. Bungee cords would be wrapped around their legs to immobilize them so they could experience the "feeling" of paralysis.

The pilot was held for fourteen second-year med students.

This seminar is now required for all University of Pennsylvania medical students. It is also a requirement for third-year nursing students at Villanova School of Nursing in Pennsylvania. The program goals include increasing knowledge of the culture, diversity, and challenges of people living with disability as well as understanding the cyclical nature of adaptation to disability or chronic illness. Participants are encouraged to identify their own biases, stereotypes, and assumptions; to educate others; and advocate for those unable to do so for themselves.

At the outset, topics relevant to living with disability are presented in a didactic and interactive way. Pairs are then randomly assigned roles of care-partner or person living with a disability. The physical limitations are reproduced in as realistic a way as possible. Pairs are assigned a series of specific tasks in the "real world" environment, such as going for lunch, using a restroom, and doing some shopping. They are told to observe their physical sensations, thoughts, and feelings. They are asked to observe how their partner behaves as well as reactions of people they encounter.

The impact is palpable in the classroom upon their return. Space does not allow me to summarize the feedback we've gotten, but it is safe to say that these learners are changed by the experience. Suddenly they encounter obstacles everywhere. "You're used to doing what you want, when you want," Malaka Jackson, a student playing the role of a disabled person, told the *Philadelphia Inquirer.* "You're not used to relying on someone else. It's not just one favor you're asking, it's lots of favors. You lose all control."

We have also adapted this program for other audiences, including corporations conducting diversity training, psychology graduate students, and other allied health professionals.

Many people comment on the courage that I, and others like me, show in the face of chronic illnesses that come into our lives and steal our self-esteem, independence, and in my case, the career I cherished. Am I courageous? Sometimes I am. Other times, I am like the Cowardly Lion in *The Wizard of Oz,* tightly clenching my tail and using it to wipe tears away.

But now, when people ask, "Alicia, what do you do?" I reply by telling them a bit about who I am, and what I do, knowing that both are not necessarily synonymous, although for some of us fortunate ones they are. I am a physician and a patient. I am an educator. I am a woman who chooses to live and give, perhaps in spite of, and perhaps because of, my journey with multiple sclerosis.

For more information: *www.conillinst.org*

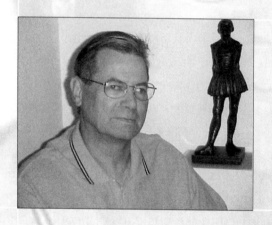

CHAPTER 3

Gardens for All

ANTHONY ZAREMBA

MY WIFE, DOROTHY, IS ONE of these naturalists who believes in organic vegetables. For seven years we had been part of a community garden in Floyd Bennett Field in Brooklyn's Gateway National Park. I used to go with her and help garden. She would pull me into the garden by a path she had made to accommodate my wheel-chair. We spent many a day together at our garden plot, and nothing beat the therapeutic, restful feeling of a day in the sun there, with me painting with my watercolors and Dorothy tending the vegetables.

But I used to see busloads of people with cerebral palsy coming there, and they couldn't do the same thing I was doing because they didn't have a special path. It was Dorothy's idea to apply for a grant, and I told her that if we received it I wanted to build accessible community garden plots not only for individuals with MS but for all people with disabilities. On July 21, 2002, my dream came true when a disability garden was dedicated in my name. ―――――――

My wife, Dorothy, and I met on a used car lot in Brooklyn, New York. Her car had actually been stolen; she was with her best friend. We had an instant connection. Needless to say, she ended up marrying me, and her best friend married my brother. We're all still best friends today.

When we were first married, the four of us would fish, play tennis, ride bikes, and play softball. There was no indication that I was sick. I was a dental technician, making great money. Plans were in place to go into business with my brother. But one day, out of the blue, Dorothy got a call from my boss. He told her, "Something's wrong with your husband. His hands are shaking; is he on drugs? Is he drinking?"

I hadn't told Dorothy about the symptoms I was experiencing. I didn't know what was wrong with me, but I didn't want to worry her. But now I couldn't hide the symptoms anymore, so I sat down with Dorothy and told her everything— about the shaking hands and the change in my eyesight and now the loss of my job. We went to a series of neurologists and finally got the diagnosis of MS.

We were pretty shaken. I was out of work and I was having physical changes that I did not understand. I didn't know what we were going to do to pay the bills. Dorothy had an idea. She had worked at a public library since she was fifteen years old. She suggested that I apply for a job there as a maintenance man. I got the job, but over time it became more and more difficult for me to do heavy maintenance repairs. I struggled with a leg brace and a cane, but fortunately I had a wonderful rapport with my supervisor, and when it became evident that I could no longer perform arduous work, he assigned me to work in the maintenance stock room. I worked at the library for over ten years and retired with a pension.

In 1999 I had a very severe exacerbation—an attack of trigeminal neuralgia— a disorder of the fifth cranial (trigeminal) nerve that causes episodes of intense, stabbing, electric shock-like pain in the areas of the face where the branches of the nerve are distributed—lips, eyes, nose, scalp, forehead, upper jaw, and lower jaw. Trigeminal neuralgia (TN) is not fatal, but it is universally considered to be the most painful affliction known to medical practice. Between 1 and 2 percent of patients with MS have TN. The cause of TN in patients with MS is a demyelinating plaque in the trigeminal nerve or brain pathways that carry messages of sensation from the face. I have never experienced such excruciating pain; I lost thirty pounds.

I had a minimally invasive neurosurgical procedure—gamma knife radio surgery—to partially damage the nerve and thus relieve the pain. The pain was gone, but the experience of the exacerbation left me emotionally drained. I started losing hope.

I'd had MS for fifteen years at that point and it had always been an uphill battle, but now I wasn't sure how much more I could take. You know, I started asking, "Why me?" And I hadn't done that before.

Once again it was Dorothy who came through. Just as she figured out the pension plan, she knew what I needed for my depression. She had read about a grant available to MS patients who wanted to help others. She looked at me, as depressed as I was, and said, "You are a true champion, Anthony. You've been battling this for so long, and you are still walking. Now, let's give hope to others." Her faith in me and her knowledge of just what to do literally saved my life.

She asked me what I thought would make a difference for others suffering. I thought about my life over the past years and knew the one diversion that had kept me going: time spent in the garden. Dorothy is one of these naturalists who believe in organic vegetables. For seven years we had been part of a community garden in Floyd Bennett Field in Brooklyn's Gateway National Park. I used to go with Dorothy and help garden. She would pull me into the garden by a path she had made to accommodate my wheelchair. I spent many a day at our garden plot, and nothing beat the therapeutic restful feeling of a day in the sun there. I would paint with my watercolors and Dorothy would tend the vegetables.

But I used to see busloads of people with cerebral palsy coming there, and they couldn't do the same thing I was doing because they didn't have a special path. I told Dorothy that if we received the grant I wanted to build accessible community garden plots not only for individuals with MS but for all people with disabilities.

My dream came true. On July 21, 2002, a disability garden was dedicated in my name.

Many of my fellow gardener volunteers from the Floyd Bennett Garden Association (FBGA) helped design and build the garden. It features twelve wheelchair-level planting stations, each ten feet by two feet by thirty inches high, arranged around the perimeter of a 400-square-foot lot. A brick pathway leading up to the garden, paved aisles between the beds, and a wide center aisle with additional planting stations provide ample space for wheelchairs to maneuver. Hanging plants attached to pulleys can be raised and lowered as needed. A wide swinging entry gate allows gardeners to enter and exit without assistance. Volunteers also installed an irrigation system and two wheelchair-level sinks for clean up. Use of machinery, plants, and garden materials were donated by FBGA, and the signage was donated by a local business. The new beds have been planted with tomatoes, cucumbers, peppers, beans, and other vegetables so that gardeners with disabilities can cultivate and harvest their crops.

Yes, I pulled myself out of the depression to create an opportunity to share the beauty of nature with other physically challenged people. At the dedication ceremony everyone kept telling me how much courage I had, how giving I was. But in my eyes, in my heart, I know who really has courage—my Dorothy. Because she believed in me with her heart and soul even when, especially when, I was ready to give up, because she believed I could rise, I did. I thank her for her love, care, and friendship.

You can visit Anthony Zaremba's Website at: *hometown.aol.com/njdotz/myhomepage/artgallery.html*

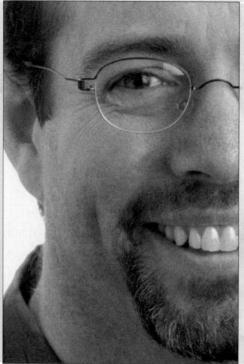

CHAPTER 4

Frank Siteman, 2003

Creating a Cure Map

ART MELLOR

I HAVE TO ADMIT THAT I WAS NOT always a very giving person, but having MS and watching others give has changed all that. _____

"We'll check your blood, but don't get your hopes up. I really think this is MS. You should go on a treatment. Do you have any questions?"

That was the verbatim delivery of my diagnosis of multiple sclerosis. Suddenly my perfect life came to a screeching halt. I was thirty-seven years old.

At the time of my diagnosis I was the chief technical officer of a high-tech company I had cofounded with a friend from MIT. I had recently sold another company that I had cofounded. It was the peak of the Internet boom, we had just finished raising $27 million in venture capital financing, we were growing like crazy, and our product was really coming together.

On the home side, I had just moved in with Debbie, the woman of my dreams, and planned to ask her to marry me later that year. I was at the top of my career, my personal life couldn't have been better, and everything was going fantastically. It looked like financial independence, personal fulfillment, and realization of my career dreams were finally within my grasp.

Sitting in the doctor's office that 14th of June 2000, all I could do was picture myself in a wheelchair (the classic "oh my God" reaction to an MS diagnosis), my girlfriend leaving me, and me unable to work, walk, or feed myself.

It was natural for me to leap to worst-case scenarios. Running a business, I did that every day. When presented with any problem it somehow helped to know what the worst-case situation might be so I could decide if it was worth spending energy on it and if so, where.

This scenario was different though. I didn't know what I could do. I didn't have the information I needed. I didn't even really know what multiple sclerosis was. Being an engineering nerd, I immediately jumped onto the Internet and searched for pages on MS. There were so many, but after a while it became clear that most were filled with the same stock descriptions of the disease or just provided links to other pages. There were a few gems in there, but they were few and far between.

Next, I went and bought all the books on MS that I could find at my local bookstore. These had some helpful descriptions of what the disease is and how it might or might not progress, but they tended to focus more on the "so you're going to be a cripple" angle rather than the "let's fix it" front.

When I complained to my new neurologist, Dr. Tim Vartanian (I had changed providers after the first did such a miserable job of presenting my diagnosis), about the lack of detailed information on the state of MS research, he gave me a number of textbooks he had used and suggested some others. I read them as quickly as I could and came to a shocking conclusion: nobody was really working on a cure for this disease in an organized and systematic fashion.

I couldn't believe this, so I set up meetings with some local MS researchers (I was lucky to be living in Boston where there are quite a few), which simply confirmed my findings.

It took me about six months to accept the fact that this wasn't just a bad dream. At that point I realized that if I wanted solutions to this problem, I would have to dedicate my life to it. I wasn't sure how, but I knew I had to find a way.

At first I thought I would quit my job and go back to school to become a researcher. Science was my first love, after all. But it occurred to me that there were many smart people already doing that and here we were with no known cause, no known cure, and a very poor understanding of what the disease even is. What was missing was the plan of attack and the centralized coordination to pull it off. My entrepreneurial background had given me extensive experience in the areas of planning and execution of plans to make things happen. Raising money, forming business alliances, creating products and processes where there were none before were all things I was good at. I figured this was where I should apply my efforts.

So I did. I quit my job and took off a few months to "decompress," then slowly began to formulate my plan of action. In the meantime Debbie and I got engaged. I wasn't sure she fully understood what she had signed up for, but I sure tried to make her understand. She said she did, and that's what mattered to me.

I started talking about my idea with Tim at my follow-up neurology appointments, and he agreed that something needed to be done to shake up the system. We began meeting regularly and our meetings resulted in the formation of the Boston Cure Project for multiple sclerosis (*www.bostoncure.org*), a nonprofit organization. Our belief is that the fastest route to a cure will come from knowing the causes of MS. To know the causes we need to have a plan of attack—what do we know already, what do we need to know, how do we go about finding it out?

We decided to create and execute that plan, a plan we call the Cure Map.

Over the course of 2001 we began setting up the infrastructure for the organization: incorporation, office space, Website, lawyer, accountant, bank account, 501(c) 3 tax-exempt status, etc. We quite literally started in a garage. A friend had been leasing an old service station to store his racecars and operate his consulting business, and he sublet on office to us at extremely low rates.

In August Debbie and I got married, and when we returned from our honeymoon I started working full-time for the organization. By the end of the year we'd hired another full-time person, Andii Briggs, as operations manager; created a Board of Directors, Board of Advisors, Scientific Advisory Board, and Pharmaceutical Advisory Board; and had a host of volunteers helping us out. In November we had our kick-off party, featuring David Lander (Squiggy from *Laverne & Shirley*) and Liane Mark (Miss Waikiki)—our first two MS celebrity endorsers.

In the year since then we've grown to four full-time staff, two part-time on-site volunteers, two part-time off-site volunteers, three consultants, 150+ on-call volunteers, and seventeen advisors of various sorts. But the most important accomplishment has been the creation of a plan that we believe will lead us to determining the causes of MS, assuming that they can be determined at all.

It has been about two and a half years since my diagnosis and my life has changed completely. I spend my days doing many of the same things I did before, but the people I interact with and the information I need to process and make decisions on are completely different. It has been extremely difficult to start my career over from scratch, building up new networks and support structures, creating another organization from the ground up in a completely different field, getting work done with volunteers rather than paid employees, and learning to raise money for a promise rather than a product. I have needed to give myself a super-quick education in biology, medicine, the health-care industry, clinical trials, and the nonprofit world. Luckily there are some good books and advisors to help.

But it has been very fulfilling in unexpected ways. Before, I mainly met people in high-tech, but MS touches the lives of people without regard to what they do, so now I'm in contact with a much wider variety of people from all walks of life. I have met doctors and accountants and mechanics and police officers and stay-at-home moms. And I have been touched by the philanthropy of those around me who have helped us build our organization. Generous contributions of money, time, and services have poured in from so many people.

And while I am ultimately doing this for purely selfish reasons—I want a cure *for me*—I find that it brings an unexpected satisfaction to me to think that what I am spending my time on may turn out to benefit so many others in a lasting and significant way. It makes those really bad days worth plowing through, knowing that our progress can make such a difference.

The Website for Art Mellor's Boston Cure organization is: *www.bostoncure.org*

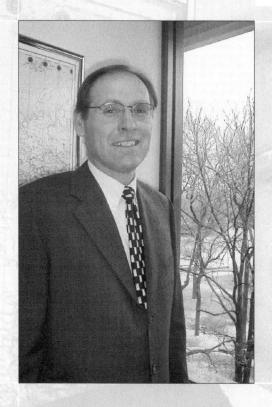

CHAPTER 5

Organizing a Team for Charity

DWIGHT RISKEY

I THOUGHT THAT AFTER TWENTY-ONE YEARS I knew everybody at Frito-Lay, but our MS 150 team, the Cheesy Riders, allowed me to meet a whole new set of people in a completely neutral, non-work-related context. Nothing could be better for building a network of strong personal connections in an organization. It also attracted the most wonderfully diverse set of participants—ethnically, functionally, hierarchically, age, and gender diverse. By its very nature, working together on this event is all about inclusion. Try it. I promise you, you will be rewarded beyond your wildest expectations.

The story goes that about 140 years ago Abraham Lincoln and a good friend had a running debate about the nature of altruism. Lincoln argued that no action is ever truly altruistic . . . that there is always, if you just dig deep enough, a selfish motive behind every generous or charitable behavior.

One day he and his friend were riding in a carriage along a rough road when they saw a litter of tiny piglets stuck helplessly in a puddle of mud. Lincoln stepped off the carriage right up to his knees in the mud to rescue the little pigs and send them on their way. As Lincoln crawled back into the carriage, a muddy mess, his friend just remarked, "I rest my case. There was no possible reward or selfish motivation behind your kind action."

Lincoln thought for a minute, and then replied, "Oh, to the contrary. I would have heard the squeals of those little creatures in my dreams."

Now, between you and me, it is not worth debating the fine philosophical points of this little story. Let's just be practical. Whether or not you believe Lincoln had a valid point, the deed was done, and it was a good deed. The piglets were saved.

I am a senior vice president at Frito-Lay. For Frito-Lay or any corporation to help support research to eradicate MS, help raise funds to support its victims— these are undeniably good, meaningful things to do. The secondary benefits like team building, improved morale, and a positive corporate culture may be considered ulterior motives. If they are, I believe we should encourage all the ulterior motives we can get.

I'm involved in the MS 150 Bike Tour, and I can tell you that my motives are anything but purely altruistic. For me and my team, it all started about two years ago when the son of an old friend asked if I would help fund his ride in the MS Bike 150. I said yes and happened to be near the finish line of the first day of the ride.

To watch my friend's son and a few hundred other riders cross that finish line was an incredibly moving experience. The thought of riding a hundred miles— well, it was just an amazing concept to me. But I noticed that there were riders my age, even older. I walk with a pretty distinct limp from my MS, but I noticed that there were a number of riders that had much tougher physical limitations than I do. Some of the riders looked as if they were in great shape; others looked, honestly, like they could afford to lose a few pounds. Suddenly, it struck me. Maybe I could ride, too.

Shortly thereafter I asked to join the team that I had supported, Se Astringo, which means commitment. But the captain wouldn't have it. She encouraged me to start my own "starter team" at Frito-Lay.

I got a bike and started riding. We had a couple of little organization meetings and an individual on our team came up with the team name Cheesy Riders—as a play on our Chester Cheetah spokescat for Cheetos. Landor, the company that designs our package graphics, has some bike riders. They offered to do a jersey design—gratis.

I tell you, the excitement was just contagious. It seemed like pretty soon everybody was talking about the Cheesy Riders.

At nearly every training ride we had a surprising number of people turn out. We had volunteers coming out of the woodwork. It wasn't just your run of the mill corporate activity, it was a MOVEMENT! It reminded me of the sixties . . . well, there weren't any drugs, but you know what I mean.

And what were the organizational benefits? Well, I'd like to emphasize three:

1. ADVENTURE STORIES. Have you ever shared a life-threatening experience with anyone? You know how different you feel about that person forever after? Well, this was not a life-threatening experience by any stretch of the imagination, but its intensity carried the same sort of emotional weight. You cannot help but feel a deep personal connection with people who share as intense an adventure as the MS 150.

   On the softer side, my wife, Cynthia, who also rode the 150 miles, calls this sort of thing "making memories." The MS 150 was a fantastic way to make a bunch of really powerful memories—with people you'd otherwise hardly known except to say hello in the hallway. I thought that after twenty-one years I knew everybody in our organization, but the Cheesy Riders allowed me to meet a whole new set of people in a completely neutral, non-work-related context. *Nothing* could be better for building a network of strong personal connections in an organization.

2. Diversity. I'm not sure why, maybe because of the socially nonthreatening nature of the activity, but the Cheesy Riders seem to attract the most wonderfully diverse set of participants. Ethnically diverse, functionally diverse, hierarchically diverse, diverse in age and gender—there is virtually no other kind of activity that I know of that can pull together such an astoundingly diverse group of employees. By its very nature it was all about inclusion.

We have a Hispanic advisory board at Frito-Lay to help facilitate Hispanic inclusion in our company culture. I serve on the board. As a part of one of the meetings, we arranged for a few of our Hispanic professionals to do a little panel Q & A about their experiences in our corporate culture.

One of our young Hispanic professionals commented on the challenges of being a woman *and* an ethnic minority. She said that the number one thing that made her feel included and connected to our company was our little Cheesy Riders team. It has been a powerful force for inclusion.

And by the way, the MS 150 is *not* just about athletes. It's not exclusionary in that way either. Although there are a few serious bike riders, the truth is, most of the Cheesy Riders had never taken anything like this type of physical challenge before.

Don't get me wrong. Everybody took the task very seriously from the fundraising, the training, to the team building. We had a team of over seventy riders, and we ended up with a team of some fifty volunteers. I think this year we'll need more volunteers, because at least half of the volunteers from last year will be riding this year!

3. Beyond Corporate. Putting this team together had very little to do with me, or really even with Frito-Lay as a big company. Frito-Lay was a sponsor, but it had a kind of loose, fairly unsupervised affiliation. I think that was an important success factor for us.

Once we got a very small wind in our sail, the Cheesy Riders were not about boring committees and taskforces. The team was a sort of living entity that thrived on its own energy. Everyone who wanted to could be a leader. There was plenty to do; none of it was a job requirement. It was kind of like a group art project—a simultaneous creative exercise. I believe it was one of the most rewarding, corporate activities that most of us had ever been involved with. And the day after the ride, I received some of the most moving notes from my team. They described it as personally rewarding, inspiring, and hugely fun.

So, I guess in closing, I'd just say I don't really care why Lincoln saved the baby pigs. The bottom line is that they're healthy, they're happy, and Lincoln feels good too.

I would encourage anyone to organize a team for a charity event. I promise you, you and your company will be rewarded beyond your wildest expectations.

Visit *redriverchallenge.ms150.org/rrc/rrc/*. For bike tours in your community, see: *www.nationalmssociety.org*

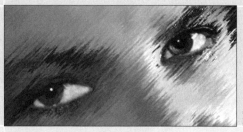

CHAPTER 6

Hal Kern

Always Be Authentic

JILL S.

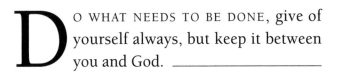

DO WHAT NEEDS TO BE DONE, give of yourself always, but keep it between you and God. _____

It was 1982. I was seventeen, a wild kid just out of high school. By day, I was a college student who wore preppy Ralph Lauren polos and couldn't decide whether to be an artist or a dental hygienist. By night, I was a party animal with glow-in-the-dark eyeshadow, who cruised around town in my restored, Super Chicken yellow Ford Falcon, my big, ratted, hair-sprayed hair barely blowing in the breeze.

One night, driving home from my last class of the day, the radio blasting the Go-Gos' "Our Lips Are Sealed," I pulled into the local self-service gas station and noticed a little old lady who seemed to be having a hard time maneuvering the nozzle. She reminded me of Ruth Gordon in *Harold and Maude*—she was probably in her late seventies or early eighties, with sweet, sparkly eyes. I thought she was adorable. I got out of the car and walked over to offer her some help. She said, "Oh, thank you, honey, I would love some help." I put the nozzle in her tank and while it was filling up we made small talk—the usual "how you doing?" "how's your day going so far?" kind of thing.

But suddenly the tone of the conversation darkened as she confided, "You know, I'm having a hard day. My husband passed away recently, and he used to be the one to do this. I'm kind of clumsy because I've got arthritis. It's so kind of you to help me out." I told her I was happy to help. Then she leaned in and said, "But it's important that you hear what I'm going to say. Are you listening?" Quietly I said, "Yeah . . ." She continued, "It's important that you continue to do good things for people, and that you continue to give unconditionally. I think you will learn a great lesson from this."

I found myself getting a little choked up. I lightly touched her arm. "It's okay," I said. She went on: "A small thing like this can be really huge. So I want you to remember something." She reached over and patted my hand. "Whenever you do a good thing, a giving thing, you mustn't talk about it. People who tell aren't giving for the right reasons; they do it because it makes them feel good, and that's not unconditional. You can tell people this story, but *real* good things are between you and God."

All I could utter was "Wow. Okay . . ."

I just stood there as she got into her car and turned on the ignition. She looked up at me and said, "Thank you so much. You made my day." Then, with a wink and one last smile, she drove away.

Standing speechless in the middle of a gas station lot, impressionable seventeen-year-old that I was, I made the most important vow of my life to a stranger I would never see again.

That was twenty years ago. Suffice to say, since that time my personal journey has been an all day/all night ticket on the "Jill Plans and God Laughs Ride of a Lifetime."

Not long after this chance encounter I left behind an art scholarship, dental school, and a job as a dental assistant to open up my own business. The economy was rockin', and busy, affluent people were happy to pay giant money for all kinds of services. "Not Enough Time" provided landscapers, house cleaners, errand runners, and dog walkers—whatever people needed. It was a huge success. Money started pouring in and I was working like crazy.

A few years later my life took a completely unexpected turn when two florist client-friends in Laguna Beach asked me to help them find someone to water plants for them for ten bucks an hour. When I asked a friend if she knew anyone for the job, she blew me away by suggesting that I do it.

I said, "No way," and reminded her that I was now earning as much money as a doctor! But without missing a beat, she said, "Yes, but you haven't learned anything."

Ouch. Way deep down, I knew she was right. So I closed up my business, keeping just a few clients, and for the next three years, every day from 7:30 A.M. to 5:30 P.M., I learned everything there was to know about plants. In time, I became an award-winning interior landscape designer, had tons of high-profile clients, and was featured in all kinds of magazines. I absolutely loved what I did. Eventually I went back to the old business, adding an interior landscaping division. Once again, it was a huge success. And I was still working like crazy.

But somehow, no matter how exhausted I was, I always honored the promise I made to that old woman at the gas station. Whenever I heard of anyone in any kind of need, I would just quietly take care of it. I'd turned into a kind of Secret Santa. And if I couldn't help, I always knew someone who could. I didn't do it because it made me feel good; I did it because it was what needed to be done.

And, just as the old woman had asked, I repeated the story of our chance encounter hundreds of times—to homeless people I'd meet, shirtless, jobless, broken hearted, whatever it was. That story just always came up. It still does. I'd always been a positive and enthusiastic person, always doing little things for other people, but after that "chance" meeting, it became a way of life for me.

And that was only the beginning. While I was busy working by day and giving to others by night, the Universe was busy working overtime to give me a gift of some heavy-duty life lessons—lessons that came in the most fascinating wrapping.

In August of 1996, my business partner and chief numbers person/money handler suggested we rethink our finances and cut out "unnecessary" expenses, which included a pricey medical insurance policy I'd had for ten years. I was always in excellent health, and in all that time, had never once been to the doctor. So we canceled the insurance immediately and decided to get a new, bare bones policy starting in January.

One night a month later, insurance-free and without a care in the world, I was entertaining a friend from out of town. When it came time to leave and she asked for driving directions back to the freeway, I said, "No problem—just follow me." She didn't see the cement truck up ahead either, blocking all lanes in both directions, trying to make an illegal three-point U-turn, but she did have a bird's eye view when I flew around the bend and plowed into that truck head on at fifty-five miles an hour. The front of my Jeep Cherokee was a disaster—even my steering wheel was bent like a taco.

I hit my head good and hard, which left my brain pretty scrambled for a while. The doctors said I had what is called "post-concussion syndrome" and that it would eventually balance out. I wished I could have gotten the same prognosis for my bank account—and that I hadn't canceled that medical insurance policy when I did.

Still scrambled, I went back to work as soon as I could. Because the left side of my brain bore the brunt of the crash, my right brain heavily overcompensated, which super-heightened my creativity. Although I hired someone to drive me around for fear that my temporary short-term memory loss might kick in at any time, I was designing the most incredibly beautiful floral and interior landscaping designs of my life. And once again I was working like crazy.

By the time the holiday season rolled around, it was Full Tilt-Boogie. I was working my brains out—whatever little I had left—eighteen hours a day, for sixty days straight. I was so completely drained and spent, that I didn't even have the energy to go to Las Vegas to spend the holiday with my parents. On Christmas Eve, after I did my last floral arrangement of the season and had a holiday bite to eat at a friend's house, I dragged myself into my apartment, threw on my favorite oversized flannel shirt and sweatpants, got up just enough strength to get a little fire going in the fireplace, collapsed onto my armchair, and feel asleep. When I woke up, I was cold and exhausted. A few tiny embers were still smoldering in the fireplace, so I walked over and put my back to the fire to get warm. When my shirt got a little too warm, I lightly pulled it away from my body and gave it a little tug, which must have sent one of those little embers right over to my shirt and given it just enough oxygen to ignite my entire back-side. I could see the reflection of that unbelievably bright light in the mirror on the wall. I went up in flames like a Roman candle.

Turns out I had third-degree burns over 23 percent of my body, and six inches of my formerly long hair was completely singed. Because the local hospital couldn't handle burns this severe, I was flown to the University Medical Center Burn Unit in Las Vegas, where I was treated for a month. At that point, because I refused to stay there another minute, my mom, who happens to be a retired nurse, set up a sterile environment at her home and took over my care.

You would think that after I slammed into a cement truck and got third-degree burns over my entire backside, I *might* have gotten the message that the Universe was trying to tell me to slow down. But noooo. I went home too soon and, surprise, I went back to work. Finally admitting to myself that I probably *was* overdoing it, I trimmed my business down to just the design, décor, and errands divisions. But somehow I was still putting in crazy hours, partly because I was trying to get out of debt from all those medical bills from the crash and the fire.

I kept that up for three years, when one day I got a call from my mom, who had recently beaten throat cancer. She said, "Jill, you're done. You need to come home." I said, "What do you mean?! I *am* home! I have a great apartment on the ocean; work is going great. Everything is wonderful!"

She pressed on. "Chuck [my dad] and I have talked it over, and we want you to come hang out with us for a while. To make the deal sweet, we'll give you an all-expenses-paid, early-inheritance year off." I kept insisting that I was fine, but she just persisted: "No, you're done." I knew that she was right. After all, I'm her kid—and by that time we had become *so* close I couldn't hide anything from her. Even the fact that my work situation wasn't actually that great and that I had just ended another failed relationship.

So I got rid of everything that wouldn't fit in a five-by-seven storage unit and drove out to Las Vegas. I loved being home with Mom and Dad. They took such great care of me. When my thirty-fifth birthday rolled around in November, I asked my best friend of twenty years to come visit. We were at the movies one night when all of a sudden I couldn't see. It was like there was a big patch of fog/smog over my left eye. My friend suggested that I might have strained my eyes from seeing way too many movies in one weekend.

The truth was, a lot of things had been going on with my body for the past two years that I hadn't told anyone about. I figured I was probably just having some residual nerve damage from the burns, or just some repercussions from everything my body had been through. Or maybe I was just getting old. My solution was to go to the chiropractor or get a massage every once in a while. The symptoms would go away and I'd feel better. I didn't know that these were things called "exacerbations" that would come and then disappear, which is why many people go undiagnosed.

I also had numbness in my hands and my feet, and one particularly fascinating whopper—I'd be walking down the street when all of a sudden my arm would jerk wildly and cramp up like I'd gotten hit in the funny bone—turning my hand into a claw. I always hoped no one saw. Sometimes I would walk like I was drunk. Sometimes my speech was a little weird, and I would feel this numbness from my trunk down to my leg.

But the loss of vision was the thing that really freaked me out. So I finally dragged myself to an eye doctor. As he was looking in my eyes, he asked me how old I was. When I said thirty-five, he got this worried look. "I absolutely see nerve damage in there. Look, you have something called optic neuritis. It might not be reversible. I suggest you go to a neurologist and get an MRI because there's a one-in-four chance that you have MS."

"WHAT?!!!! I have WHAT?!!!!" I had no idea what MS was, but I knew it couldn't be good. The look on my mom's face told the whole story. The doctor decided against giving me glasses or an eye patch or anything. He said "Look, just come back and see me in thirty days, and let's see what happens."

Within those next thirty days I went from "can't see" to "really can't see" to "totally blind" (in that one eye). My vision went from 20/20 to 20/60. Every single morning before I opened my eyes, I prayed. And I prayed. I would say to myself "Okay, c'mon. It's got to be better . . . It's GOT to be better!" Wouldn't you know, when I went back to see the eye doctor a month later, my vision was miraculously back to 20/20. He said, "I don't know who you are, but I don't ever want to see you again. You had optic neuritis, and now, you don't! Good for you! Go have a good life! But you still might want to get that MRI." Mom and I left the office and did a little happy dance in the parking lot.

I didn't tell anyone that I was having all those other symptoms—including the phenomenal fatigue. And of course I was doing everything wrong for someone in a full-blown exacerbation. In fact what I did would have sent most people to the hospital. I went to the gym every day, used the Jacuzzi (which you're *never* supposed to do), spent forty-five minutes a day on the treadmill, then the exercise bike, then sat in the dry sauna, then went home and passed out. I might not have been officially diagnosed with MS, but I was definitely an official lunatic. And I still hadn't gone to a neurologist or gotten that MRI.

I had to keep myself busy because something told me I wasn't going back to Laguna. I was determined to get to work, so I continued to send out resumes, but I just had to find out what I had. So, in full-tilt survival mode, I got onto the Internet and started reading everything I could about MS. There it was in black and white—everything I'd been experiencing for the past two years: the fatigue, the numbness, even the weird arm thing. When I read about the neurological spinal stuff, where you can get a strange electrical shock through your body when you try to put your chin to your chest, I was pretty well convinced. It couldn't be a coincidence that I had all these symptoms. But one little part of my brain still clung to the thought that it might all just go away.

I certainly didn't slow down. I got a job selling the showroom of a popular high-end hotel and started working insane hours again. Eighteen- to twenty-hour days were not uncommon. At first the MS was manageable; it was always at the back of my mind, but I was completely driven to get on with my life and not have a disease. So I kept going. And going.

Then, after a few months at that ridiculous pace, I got incredibly sick. All the symptoms flared up big time. I got so sick that I finally went to a neurologist. He wanted to give me a spinal tap. After twelve failed tries at extracting some fluid from my spine, I couldn't take the pain anymore. Even my third-degree burns didn't hurt this much! I said, "I've got to get out of here! You have got to stop!"

I had moved out of my parents' house and was living with a friend who just happened to have a friend who was a top cancer researcher at the University of

Utah, who just happened to go fly fishing with a top MS doctor. By this time, my equilibrium was so bad that I couldn't even lift my head up off the pillow without heaving my guts out. Getting out of bed to go the bathroom often became an all-day event. Before I knew it, my friend had put me on a plane alone to Utah to see the neurologist. Two hours after landing, I was officially diagnosed. Not only did I have MS, but I had it full-tilt—with spectacular lesions. I had no idea what "spectacular lesions" were, but I could tell this wasn't exactly a compliment. He remarked that anyone seeing my MRIs and looking at my history would think I was in a wheelchair. The fact that I was vertical and functioning was, to him, "just amazing."

The diagnosis finally made, I thought my whole world would stop. What would happen to me? What would I do if I couldn't work?! I made a deal with the doctor: I promised to keep my workday down to ten hours and he told me everything I needed to know about the ABC drugs. He sent me home, and I went back to work.

These days I work at one of the leading destination management/entertainment and modeling companies in Las Vegas, with some of the nicest people around. It's a very "MS friendly" place because a few of my colleagues know or are related to people who have MS. Mornings are usually the hardest—a bit like getting the ol' Spruce Goose off the tarmac. I just drag my sorry ass out and somehow get to work. I certainly have days where my body has plans of its own. But once everything starts feeling good again, I'm back in business, selling, producing, creating, being a part of a great team.

So I just keep going. And giving. And praying. I keep my mind so busy that I don't pay much attention to what's going on in my body. The exacerbations come more frequently than I would like them to, but I just move through them with as much grace as I possibly can. I learned that from my mom. She's been absolutely amazing, the strongest female I've even seen. She's gone through so much in her life with such sheer grace and authenticity—and that's what I want most in my life—to be 100 percent authentic and to do everything from a place of love and grace. I would love to have that be my legacy.

Lucky for me, authenticity and grace seem to run in my family. During World War II, I'm told, my grandfather, an affluent dentist, used to make a habit of picking up the checks for soldiers dining nearby. My dad, a rough old Cajun and proud marine from the bayous of Louisiana, was apparently something of an angel to a bunch of alcoholics and drug users—a fact we only learned after he died. So what that old woman and I didn't know is that there's something of a family tradition to helping—and keeping it secret. And I certainly haven't forgotten my part. I organized a group of women in Las Vegas that I like to call the Angel Mafia. They are all busy women involved with the world of entertainment. You'll never know their names, but whenever any of us sees or hears of someone in need—we've helped single moms pay their electric bills, found housing for women coming out of rape crisis centers, bought eyeglasses for children, given rides to moms who didn't have cars, fundraised for homeless children, given makeovers to recovering alcoholics reentering the work place—all we have to do is pick up the phone and help is on the way. We just get it there, we do it, and we go.

Since I'm involved in the MS community in a very public way, I get calls all the time from people who have been touched in some way by this disease. Whether they just got diagnosed, or they know someone who just got diagnosed, or they care for someone with MS, whatever they want to discuss, I'm always happy to talk with them—and I'm very open about my own experience. When we talk or meet, I'm always sure to tell them I understand what they are going through, reassure them that their symptoms are "normal," and give them psychological support for all the weird thoughts you can have with a disease like this (like, Why would my husband want to stay with me now when I am not a whole person?).

When you're diagnosed with something this unpredictable, you have to have someone to talk to or some safe place to go—whether you're having difficulty trying to inject yourself in the leg with medicine, or don't know which doctor to go to, how to manage your symptoms, or anything else that might come up. And something always comes up. So I just try to provide a safe place where people can vent, ask, explain, or share so they don't feel alone. I'm so grateful that I can be there for them, because I know how scary this thing is—I know exactly where they're coming from, because I've been there. I'm still there.

Sometimes we get to the gas station story. I'll say, "I can give you a 100 percent guarantee that you can fix the depression you are experiencing, but it only works if you don't tell a soul! It will change everything in your world." And we take it from there.

As for where I'm going, well, I still just suit up and show up—and wherever life takes me, I go. Somehow over the years, however—since the car accident and the fire and the MS and everything since and in between—I've learned to take a few quiet minutes every day to just enjoy life. I'll sit up on a rock and watch the snow fall on Red Rock Canyon, or look at my little puppy's bearded mug, dance with my friend Joe Clark in the kitchen, or watch little kids with chunky legs run through the park. And I still think about that woman in the gas station and her sweet, beautiful face. Who knows—she could very well have been one of God's little "worker bees" who are out there, all over the world, just spreadin' the love.

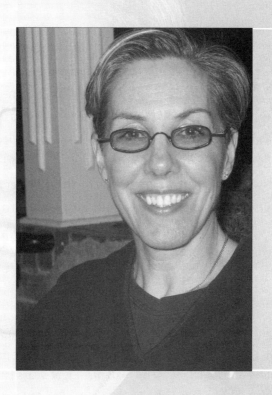

CHAPTER 7

*If You Follow Your Heart and Use Your
Mind, You Can Achieve Anything*

KATHLEEN WILSON

WHEN THE DOCTOR'S JOB IS DONE and the nurse's job is done, when the support group is over, it's critical to know we have somewhere to go. Through MSWorld (www.msworld.org) we are never alone; we always have somewhere to go to find information, share experiences, and meet wonderful people. People newly diagnosed with MS can find support and discover that MS is a manageable disease. And we all can learn from each other how to live our lives re-creating, rediscovering, and rejoicing in all that we can do. ⎯⎯⎯⎯⎯⎯⎯⎯⎯⎯

I was diagnosed with MS in 1995. I was single, thirty-seven and an artist living a very active life in Greece when, bam, the diagnosis put me into a wheelchair and sent me back home to live with my parents. Eight years later I can see that I was given an incredible opportunity to change my life, but back then I felt that I'd been condemned. The despair was devastating.

Very soon after my diagnosis I learned firsthand how isolating MS can be and how difficult it can be to get information and support. The first three months were especially hard. Many, many nights I found myself up at 3 A.M., wondering, "What am I going to do with my life? I don't even have a life." It was so hard to imagine starting over. I had loved my life as an artist, and I knew that from now on everything was going to be different. What kept me going, I think, was my strong belief that there was something important for me to do in this life. I would just have to discover what it was.

Six weeks after I returned home, my mom asked if there was anything in this world that I could possibly want that would make my life better. I'm not sure where the answer came from but it was immediate and sure: a computer. I was up and ready to go within the hour, and we came home that day with my first real computer.

With the intense fatigue I was experiencing at the time, it took a few months to get everything set up and to get online. But once I did, once I brought the world into my home, I knew that this was exactly what I needed to be doing. Relatively little information about MS was available online back then. The few chat rooms and message boards there were offered little comfort, and much of the information appeared unreliable. I wanted to know what MS was and how others were living with it. I wanted to develop strategies for re-creating my own life. I wanted that sense of belonging that comes from sharing a few words with someone else who knows what it is like to walk the same steps. Not finding what I was looking for, I decided to start my own chat room for people and families coping with MS. I started it for me, really, to help me find the support I most wanted. Little did I know that I was on my way toward fulfilling my destiny.

As soon as I started connecting with other people with MS through the Internet, I knew that I had to take this further. Armed with little other than a masters degree in mental health counseling, I started MSWorld, Inc. (*www.msworld.org*).

Today the MSWorld Website receives over 20,000 visits per day from people struggling to understand this disease and ways to cope with it. We are linked to medical Websites all over the world that report on the latest breakthroughs in MS, and we offer all kinds of support via message boards, chats, email groups, book reviews, guest hosts, and a variety of other resources. We are also the official online chat and message board for the National MS Society.

At MSWorld our motto is "Wellness is a state of mind." We offer people a place of belonging—a place where they can learn to deal with the emotional intricacies of living with MS and get information and support so that they can get on with their lives. One of the greatest benefits I've received from MSWorld is that I finally have a place to put my disease. Whenever I have questions or need support, I have a place to go. My MS doesn't have to take up so much space in the rest of my life. I'm not as dependent on people who know even less about this disease than I do for gathering information and getting my questions answered. Having this kind of access is empowering in so many ways, not least of which is that I can participate as an equal with my health team, making informed decisions about my own treatment and care.

Recently, I went to an MS clinic to treat a flare-up. The results came back on a Friday afternoon. The doctor told me, "Well, it looks like you've gone secondary-progressive with your MS and we want to put you on Novantrone. When you get home, find an oncologist, call me, and we'll get started." Needless to say, I left her office devastated. It was like being newly diagnosed all over again. I had no idea what Novantrone was and had been so stunned by her diagnosis that I just didn't have the strength to ask.

As soon as I got home, I got online and checked the Website's message boards, and sure enough, I had information on Novantrone within the hour. I learned that the drug was used to treat progressive MS and certain types of cancer. Somehow I felt in my heart that this just wasn't what I needed at this time.

By Monday I was feeling better and knew what I needed to do. I sought out two different neurologists, a specialist at the Mayo Clinic and a local neurologist, for a second opinion, and both said "no way" to the Novantrone. Having access to MSWorld saved me so much anxiety. I was able to seek out the information I needed and move forward with a more informed and realistic perspective.

The Website is currently run by thirty-two volunteers worldwide, all diagnosed with MS, all of whom have been positively affected by their ability to help others. In fact, many of the people who have volunteered at MSWorld have taken flight with dreams of their own. Some have published books, others have learned Website design, and many have started doing public speaking in an effort to help others with MS live better lives. Susan Zachary, our vice president and Web administrator, is a perfect example. She was one of a handful of people in the first online chat meeting. She says, "The minute I got in the room, it was like coming home. I was talking with people who understood what I was saying. I could talk freely."

Susan helped us build our site, one of the most user-friendly Websites on the Internet, not because she has a degree in Web design but because she had an overwhelming desire to help others. Yes, she has MS, but her passion for building this site and her desire to help others was bigger than her disease. She took the time to read books, talk to programmers, and learn everything necessary to create and maintain our wonderful home online. And now she runs her own Web consulting business out of her home.

The rewards of our work are endless. I receive emails all the time from people who depend on the site as a kind of lifeline. One woman emailed me from a nursing home to let me know how important MSWorld is to her. At forty-nine, surrounded by people who are in their eighties, she was experiencing extreme isolation and depression. "It's a really difficult time for me. I recently learned about MSWorld and it is wonderful to know it is there." I emailed her back to see if there is any possible way that she can join us and work on the Website.

I still struggle to walk and see. I have a burning sensation in my right foot that never subsides, blurry vision that comes and goes, and weakening legs that make me more dependent on my scooter every day. And I've learned to live one day at a time, knowing that at any time I might return to the condition I was in when I was first diagnosed. Each morning I strive to revive the spirit of faith that a permanent cure will come along to help me and others like me, who have had to learn to give away parts of us—both mentally and physically—every day. This is the nature of having MS and at times the sadness is overwhelming. But through my work with MSWorld I know that my experiences are making a difference for others. And that's all the proof I need that each of us matters, that if you follow your heart and use your mind, you can achieve anything.

See Kathleen Wilson's Website: *www.msworld.org*

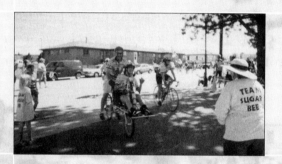

CHAPTER 8

Focusing on Wellness

KELLY WALKER-HALEY

T HE LACK OF CONTROL I FELT being diagnosed with MS was the most frustrating part for me. But there was also such a reality check; what are we really in control of anyway, besides our beliefs and how we choose to live each moment? _____

A long time ago, before I was ever diagnosed with MS, I went for a long run to let out some energy, and during the run the thought flashed through my mind that some day I was not going to be able to run away from my problems. In some mystical way, I think I was preparing myself for living with MS.

An exercise physiologist and aerobics instructor working on my masters in exercise, physiology, and wellness at Colorado State University, my entire being centered on wellness. I also worked at the university placing students in internships across the country and loved sharing my enthusiasm with them. So what does a person with a passion for wellness do when she is diagnosed with MS and confined to a wheelchair, can't teach aerobics at the health club, and can't go out and run?

The first thing she does is change her perspective. I contacted our local MS chapter for support and information. It so happened they had been trying to organize an exercise class and hadn't been successful, so I started a chair aerobics program. Some of my students from the university came over to help. If someone couldn't move their legs or even upper body very well, they would help with passive range-of-motion exercises.

My brothers, my husband, and my sister-in-law started a team for the MS Bike Tour and named it Team Sugar Bee—that's what my brother used to call me when we were growing up. Their shirts were bright yellow with black stripes, so we actually looked like a bunch of bumblebees! Team Sugar Bee grew each year. Colleagues, friends, and cousins joined the team; I would go and cheer them on. My parents even started a rest stop—The Bee Stop—with relatives and friends giving out water, food, and mostly love.

As grateful as I was for their efforts and the funds they were raising, I grew tired of being on the sidelines. Then my brother Eric told me about a grant for people with MS, and I said, "If I win, I would like to see about getting a tandem bike so I can ride with you guys."

After getting the grant, I did some inquiring and discovered Angletech—a bike shop in Woodland Park, Colorado, specializing in tandem recumbent bikes! I let them know I had no use of my legs but had strong arms. Calvin Clark at Angletech knew just what to do.

He designed an arm-crank bike for my husband, Jack, and me. The bike is amazing. It's almost like sitting in a chair—my legs are straight out in front—and I have an arm crank. I can sit and pedal with Jack. He does most of the work; he even steers.

The first time we tested the tandem, we went up to Horsetooth, some foothills right by our house. As we rode, I remember shouting, "This is incredible." I hadn't been up there since we used to hike. I felt like a bird, so free. It was like I was back in the driver's seat.

We started riding in the MS 150 on that bike. The first year, I had to train hard, about four months, but it was worth it. We only biked forty miles, but I was so psyched that it felt like we had done the entire 150.

This year, our eighth, we have three goals:

- to have 130 Team Sugar Bees
- for Jack and me to go at least twenty miles
- to continue to raise funds, awareness, and hope for those challenged with MS.

I'm in a wheelchair but I continue to move, and my hope is that others with MS find ways to do the same. I've got a mini arm-crank that I don't use enough, but I do lift five-pound weights, and I have a recumbent bike that I ride in the house. I usually have to hold my left leg and help it a little bit. I made myself a deal a long time ago; I can only watch my favorite soap, *General Hospital,* if I'm being productive, so I get on that bike Monday through Friday.

At my ten-year high school reunion people were reminiscing and someone asked, "Who was the first woman to letter nine times at Alameda?" I thought about the irony of life, laughed, and shouted, "ME!" with joy and pride.

The way I see it, it took me getting ill to get well.

I really relate to the saying "Life is 90 percent attitude and 10 percent situation." Sure, we face challenges living with MS, but it's our choice to be angry and bitter and think of ourselves as ill or to lead our lives centered on wellness— love, laughter, and maybe, maybe even riding a tandem!

For more information visit: *www.angletechcycles.com*

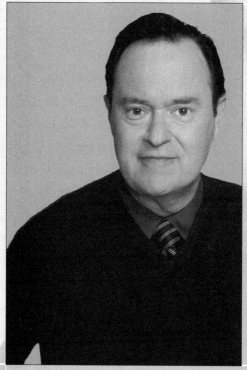

CHAPTER 9

Chris McPherson, 2002

Coming Out About MS

DAVID L. LANDER

P ERHAPS YOU KNOW ME BEST for my portrayal of Squiggy, the greasy neighbor with the spit-curl hair in the 1970s hit television series *Laverne & Shirley*. Or you may have seen me in *Who Framed Roger Rabbit?*, *A League of Their Own, Used Cars,* or *The Man with One Red Shoe.* Well, I've taken on another role in my career—I'm playing myself for the first time—it's the role I was born to play.

By telling my story I hope I can make a difference in somebody's life. I almost feel as if it's my duty to be a National Ambassador for the MS Society. When you've been "anointed" with this disease, you owe it to your fellow MS-ers—to the people in your club—to tell your story. ————————

On the set of *Conan the Destroyer* in 1983, I developed a terrible flu. I returned to the United States and immediately noticed that things were different about me. It seemed now they were building the curbs a lot higher. I experienced balance problems, difficulty holding objects and walking.

It was shortly after the final episode taping of *Laverne & Shirley* that I started to notice subtle physical problems such as numb fingers and limbs, vertigo, and difficulty with balance.

Like everyone with MS, there were clues that something was wrong with me, but nothing added up as remarkable. Symptoms appeared and disappeared as if by magic, slowly, little by little, inch by inch. I would step in holes that were not there, trip on cracks in the sidewalk, or watch a drink slip through my hands twice in one night without feeling it leave my fingertips.

It seemed like my body was out of sync, like a badly dubbed Hercules picture. I could no longer trust it to follow the simplest instructions. On some days, crossing streets and climbing curbs became a challenge. On other days I would be okay. I knew something wasn't right, I just didn't know what it was called, if it was serious, or if it would ever go away.

It was like living on a fault line. I knew a quake was coming, but I didn't know when it would erupt or how big the quake would be.

On the days my body didn't listen, I told myself it was just one of those days. But I didn't know what "one of those days" meant; nothing hurt, my body just wasn't working like it should. Then, without warning, I'd feel normal again. But, one morning I woke and couldn't move my legs.

Within days my doctor had the answer.

When I was still emerging from a fog of anesthesia, Kathy, my wife, and the neurologist stood as unsteady blurs at my bedside and delivered the news. "You have multiple sclerosis." The words sounded strange. I repeated them silently. It was unlikely that I would be able to walk again, the doctor said, and if I did, it wouldn't be for long. High doses of steroids might help in the short term. (Back then, there were no ABCR treatments available.) But in the end, the only thing I could count on was that the disease would progress. I would get worse.

My legs lay still, completely numb from the spinal tap. The information the doctor had just given me was not sinking in. It hovered in the air, separate and incomprehensible. Instead, worst-case scenarios circled through my mind. I saw

Raymond Burr in *Ironside* in a wheelchair. I turned away from the doctor and looked out the window of my room, which was in a wing of private rooms on the top floor of one of the towers at Cedars Sinai Hospital. I could see only blue sky and the silhouette of another hospital tower. The doctor droned on about all the horrible things I would look forward to, and I thought, "Talk about bedside manner! Frankly, Doctor, I am not impressed."

Three days later, I got out of my hospital bed and walked to the bathroom. I remember laughing and thinking, "I've had this disease for three days, and already I'm doing it wrong." Later I learned that I had the relapsing-remitting type of MS, hence the sudden attacks and remissions.

After being diagnosed, I thought about going public. But it took just one experience to change my mind. One day while waiting for an audition, I overheard a receptionist tell a caller that the role I was up for had already been filled. Puzzled, I asked why I hadn't been told that the part had been offered to someone else.

"Oh, it's still open," the receptionist replied. "It's just that that was Richard Pryor's agent. Pryor has multiple sclerosis. Can you believe his agent thinks he could do this part?"

I decided then and there to remain silent about my condition. I look back on the decision nineteen years later and still think it was the right one.

I tried to keep working but went to great lengths to keep my illness a secret. I did a few shows in the late nineties, like *Nash Bridges* and *L.A. Heat,* but my worst fears came true. As hard as I tried, I just could not keep up the charade. In *L.A. Heat,* I played an accountant who ran everywhere. I ran through bullets. I ran after cars. It was ridiculous. My double did most of the running, except once when I somehow—don't ask me how—did the running. The director was impatient and asked that I run a little faster. Well, I did and fell flat on my face. The same thing happened in *Nash Bridges.* My character ran everywhere. In one scene, when I was thrown through a plate glass window, I had to get up and run, avoiding pushcarts as I went. Run. Run. Run. Bang. Splat. Pushcart hits the Dave. Head hits the pavement. Everyone thought I was dead.

I wouldn't tell my producers why I would sometimes lose my balance in rehearsals. I'd say I'd hurt my back in a car accident so I couldn't do any running. Once I was rehearsing for a play in Chicago and the producers could tell I was insecure in what I was doing. My balance was wavering. They brought me into the office to talk about my "problem." They thought I was an alcoholic. I said I was! I was actually willing to allow them to think I was an alcoholic so I wouldn't lose my job. I thought, "How low could I stoop?"

For the first six years I didn't even share my diagnosis with my longtime friend Michael McKean, who played my best bud, Lenny, on *Laverne & Shirley.* I didn't want that to become part of our relationship.

In 1999, Penny Marshall, who played Laverne on *Laverne & Shirley,* called and asked me whether I was fighting MS. She'd heard a rumor from a movie producer whose daughter had the disease that I might be suffering from it as well.

Marshall told me that this producer was planning to have a dinner to benefit MS research and wanted to honor me, if I did indeed have the disease. I was shocked that someone had uncovered my secret. After talking with Kathy and Natalie, my daughter, I decided to go public.

In their June 14, 1999 issue, *People* magazine wrote an article about my struggle called "Out of Hiding." They decided to play up the courage angle. That was funny to me because I think of a firefighter going into a burning building to save a baby as someone with courage, not an actor posing as a drunk to save his career.

But it does take courage to "come out." Whether it is issues relating to work, relationships, privacy, whatever, the isolation is the same. After the *People* article, someone wrote me a letter that said, "Dear Dave, Welcome to the club." I often think about that letter. MS really is a club that none of us wanted to join, but here we are, and there is comfort in knowing we are not alone.

I hope I can make a difference in somebody's life, to really talk to people who are going through the same fears I was going through. These days I almost feel as if it's my duty to be a National Ambassador for the MS Society. When you feel as if you've been anointed with this disease, you owe it to your fellow MS-ers—to the people in your club—to tell your story.

In a way it feels tremendously liberating. I hope that others who are contemplating "coming out" will relate to my story.

For more of David's story, see his book *Fall Down Laughing: How Squiggy Caught Multiple Sclerosis and Didn't Tell Nobody,* J. P. Tarcher, 2000, and visit his Website at *www.davidlander.com.*

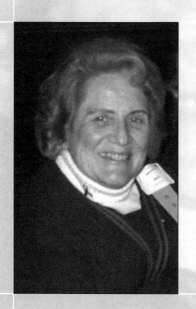

CHAPTER 10

Make Your Life Count

JEAN GRISWOLD

F OR YEARS I WAS PLAGUED with strange symptoms— numbness, acute pain, loss of balance, and lots of falls. These were finally diagnosed as MS. I'll never forget how surprised I was when dear old Dr. McClenahan, our family physician, came to our door, little black medical bag in hand, and said, "Sit down." Instead of his stethoscope, out of his bag he pulled an orchid. It was his way of trying to soften the news that I had multiple sclerosis. He added, "Now, don't go to the library and look it up." But, of course I did. I realized I'd received a life sentence, but I wasn't about to let MS hold me back.

For thirty-seven years I've struggled with the increasingly frustrating ravages of this disease. For the last ten years I have been unable to walk or to even stand. I can't even get from my bed to my wheelchair without a Hoyer lift. Yet I still go to work every day because I have a dream and am still living it. My work of providing care to the homebound has helped 60,000 people. What could be better than that? _____

My high school yearbook said: "She'll take the world by storm with her stirring speeches on business reform!" I guess my dream showed even then. As early as ten, picking apples from the tree in our backyard and selling them on the street corner, I knew I wanted to have my own business. In college I studied business law and labor relations and later earned my masters in personnel and guidance. But as interested as I was in business, when I married a minister I discovered there was a lot more to life. I knew then and there that I wanted to help people.

By the time my youngest son left home for college, fourteen years after my diagnosis, I was really beginning to confront my physical limitations, but I wasn't about to let MS hold me back. I decided I wanted to get back into business. I applied for a position with a company handling placements and gave as a personal reference my best friend, Jane, who told them, "She does very well for someone with multiple sclerosis."

You could practically hear the door slam in my face. I wasn't even in the running. As *Forbes* magazine later wrote about this turning point in my life, "She couldn't get a job, so she created one."

As I thought about what I might do to help people, I immediately thought of a close friend—a member of my husband's former congregation—who had died tragically from lack of care. I knew I couldn't let this kind of thing go on without trying to help. I figured everybody who's ill, disabled, elderly, or infirm needs someone, if only to do the little things like picking up a pair of glasses that have dropped to the floor just out of reach. Or to change a burned-out light bulb so they are not left in the dark. The kind of services that allow people to stay safely in their own homes, rather than being relegated to nursing homes.

So I decided to start a business to provide such a service, a business that would bring together my two longtime dreams—of being of service *and* an entrepreneur. I began recruiting seminary students and other caring people who could go into people's homes to provide the kind of help our elderly friend had been seeking.

If we were going to succeed, I knew I'd have to give it my undivided attention. To start and grow any business takes a lot of work and sacrifice, especially when you do it with almost no money. I gave up practically everything. Vacations were definitely out. I neglected family, friends, hobbies. I even gave up sleep for brain-storming and wee-small-hours conferences. Business became a part of every meal, every family gathering, and every waking hour. It took over my life, then my husband's life, then my son's, and now my daughter-in-law's, too.

And it all started at my dining room table. From there it took over the living room, and then we enclosed the porch. As more and more people came to us for help, we kept adding phones and desks and people. Thus began what is now known as Griswold Special Care, the largest privately owned nonmedical home care company in America, with seventy-five offices in sixteen states, and opera-tions in Mexico and South Korea. Despite being confined to a wheelchair because I cannot walk or even stand, I continue to oversee the day-to-day operations of the company. Griswold Special Care has become my arms and legs for reaching out with loving care to so many in need of help.

We've been at it for twenty years now and have helped more than 60,000 indi-viduals and families. As my husband says, "You manage to do the impossible. It just takes you longer."

The financial health of the company has allowed me to establish the Special Care Foundation, which provides home care for those who cannot afford it, and to provide a grant to establish the Griswold Special Care Wellness and Education Center in Philadelphia, which is run by the National MS Society Greater Delaware Valley Chapter. The center provides a host of programs, including exercise and education classes to help enhance the lives of people with MS, such as yoga, nutrition classes, tai chi, balance, coordination, and strengthening exercises. When I hear remarks like, "Wellness has come to have a whole new meaning for me—physically, emotionally, and spiritually, these programs have altered my overall sense of myself," it makes all my hard work worthwhile.

I have received many awards and been featured on national television and in magazines, all of which has been very satisfying, but the real reward is in knowing that Griswold Special Care has been such a blessing to so many.

I dreamt of becoming an entrepreneur and of helping others. Having MS did not stop me. For those of you who have MS, or any other limitation, I offer this challenge:

Don't focus on what you have lost (or may lose).
Focus instead on your abilities and possibilities.
Make the most of what you still have and can do.

When you become discouraged and are tempted to give up, what you need is not something to make your life easier but something that will give your life *purpose*.

And finally, find someone or something to love. It is in giving that you receive. No matter what adversity or handicap may come your way, if you have love, there will always be new and creative ways to make your life count.

Jean Griswold can be reached through her Website: *www.home-care.net/index.html*

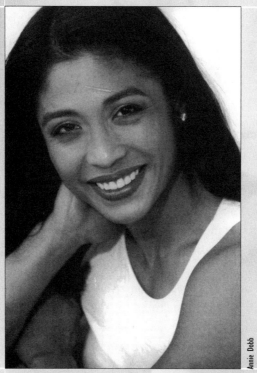

CHAPTER 11

Annie Dobb

Anything Is Possible

MARIE L. STALLBAUM

I F WE BELIEVE IN OURSELVES and our ability to live well, if we have the determination and perseverance to achieve our personal goals, anything is possible. Yes, multiple sclerosis is an unpredictable disease . . . but that's life. _____

To say I led an active life before multiple sclerosis would be an understatement. At age three I was placed in ballet, tap, jazz, acrobatics, and swimming and diving classes. When I was nine, my parents decided they couldn't continue to drive my two brothers and me all over the Chicagoland area for our extracurricular activities so we all had to choose the one we liked best. I decided to specialize in gymnastics.

Several years later, just a week before a state meet, I sustained a left knee injury, which required total knee reconstruction. The doctors said I would never be able to do gymnastics again. I didn't listen. With sheer determination, I rehabilitated my knee and eventually earned a gymnastic scholarship to the University of Wisconsin in Madison. Just before entering the NCAA scene, I had to have surgery on my right knee. Then, after competing in the NCAA for two years, I sustained a right arm fracture, which required surgical intervention. At that point my gymnastic career came to an end.

Little did I know that these experiences were simply teaching me the perseverance and determination I would so dearly need to deal with MS.

I focused on my nursing studies and became a neonatal intensive care nurse.

I enjoyed the NICU so much that I eventually went into management. The job came with a lot of responsibilities, and I typically put in twelve-hour days. Then I'd go do my workouts.

In June 1994, I started getting headaches, dizziness, double vision, and fatigue. Because I was having new eyeglasses made at the time, I attributed the symptoms to eyestrain. I figured I was just tired and that if I just found time to rest, the symptoms would subside. Even as a healthcare professional, I ignored all the signs and symptoms that something was seriously wrong. I had the glasses remade four times, but the symptoms lasted all summer. My doctor diagnosed migraine headaches.

Months later, the symptoms still persisting, I consulted an ophthalmologist, and he sent me to a neuro-opthalmologist who diagnosed me with MS. I barely even knew what those initials stood for given that my specialty was with infants, but I knew it was a disease that had no cure. I was scared and confused and had no idea how much grieving I'd have to do. I figured I was going to end up in a wheelchair in just a couple of weeks. For me, a person whose life happiness depended upon fitness, this was a death sentence.

The neuro-opthalmologist tried to keep me cheered. He told me to "just keep living your life as you always do" and to come back in two weeks. So that's what I did. I made my follow-up appointment then headed straight to the gym to work out my frustrations. I worked out as if nothing had changed—pumping weights, running, sweating, determined to show my body the diagnosis was a huge mistake. But working out was futile. I left the gym feeling weak and overwhelmingly fatigued.

Then someone suggested I get a second opinion. In November 1994, I saw a second neurologist. After evaluating my test results he said he could not officially diagnosis me with MS. Of course I was just in remission, but at the time I didn't know that. I just felt this huge relief. I told myself I didn't have MS and never would.

A few months later, my symptoms reappeared, along with complete vision loss in my left eye. That's when I was officially diagnosed with MS. I was hospitalized immediately and put on steroid therapy.

The first question I asked my neurologist was, "I don't drink, I don't smoke, I exercise, I try to eat right, why me?" He explained that this disease does not discriminate. Apparently not. But soon enough I recovered my eyesight and my symptoms started to go away. I was still in the hospital, so I found a stationary bike on the unit and the medical staff allowed me to ride for twenty minutes . . . max. I was also able to do push-ups and sit-ups in my hospital room with discretion.

Once again, I was determined to beat this thing! I committed to eating a totally clean diet, training more intensely, and doing more cardio, but the results were the same. Every time I worked out I'd be down for three days due to the over-whelming fatigue. It took several setbacks but eventually I learned that I couldn't force my body to be well. I had to listen to it, take responsibility for learning about the disease process, maintain a kind of physical balance that would inspire me to better myself, and just continually search for ways to nurture my spirit and my soul.

In 2001, I decided to compete in fitness at the Las Vegas Bodybuilding, Figure and Fitness Classic. I vowed to get into shape, but this time I would do it the smart way. During training I listened to my body and respected its limits. I just did the best I could. It felt great to be doing what I loved.

All the hard work paid off, because I became the Las Vegas Open Fitness champion! Standing onstage receiving that first place trophy, I knew without a doubt that *anything* is possible, regardless of life's adversities. Here are some general fitness pointers for anyone looking to relieve MS symptoms:

1. Always start by getting an evaluation by a health care professional and learning about the effects of MS on your body.

2. Under the supervision of your health care professional, formulate an exercise plan. Living with MS may redefine what exercise is to you. Just take a deep breath, relax, and remain flexible about the different exercise options that might be best for you. Work together to come up with various modalities that will fit into your lifestyle, whether it is working with a physical therapist to incorporate movement from a sitting position, or hydrotherapy, yoga, Pilates, NIA, or training for a fitness competition.

3. Learn some relaxation techniques. Breathing exercises, relaxation CDs/tapes, stretching techniques, massage, or even reading a book can all be great for relaxing your body and mind. Breathing techniques in particular can help circulate oxygen throughout your system and assist you in achieving a relaxed state.

4. Stretch. Good stretching exercises will allow you to increase overall flexibility, which will help with agile movements such as getting out of bed; moving to and from your wheelchair; improved balance with a walker; or when incorporated in a weight training regimen, preventing injuries, building strength, and avoiding muscle soreness.

5. Find a nutritional balance that works best in your lifestyle. Educate yourself in eating a balance of nutrients in moderation. Your body requires carbohydrates, proteins, and fats to run efficiently. Do not deprive yourself of your favorites; instead, learn to have proportionate servings, i.e., have a piece of cake, not the whole cake. Dr. George Blackburn, associate director of nutrition at Harvard Medical School, states, "It's not what you do for eight days, it's what you do for eight years." A nutritionally sound foundation will improve your overall

demeanor and will assist your therapies to work efficaciously. The human body is a phenomenal machine. A great analogy I like to share is if you owned a Lamborghini, you would not fuel it with low-grade gasoline. Your system deserves first-rate nutrients to run at the top of its game. Health is our wealth. Our bodies are our temples. No one can take that away from us.

6. Listen to your body and treat it with respect. Fatigue—deep, deep fatigue—is a common symptom in MS. MS fatigue is difficult to put in words, but what I experience can best be called "train wreck" fatigue. I often experience fatigue after a long day at work, but when "train wreck" fatigue sets in, I know not to push the envelope. It can be incredibly frustrating, but it's not worth expending energy you don't have with frustration. If you are experiencing fatigue it is very important to determine the underlying cause—i.e., depression, overwork, sleep disorders, stress, or other medical conditions. Only once the underlying issues are identified can they be effectively treated.

7. And finally, always be cognizant, even in this area of your life, that it's a learning process.

Listen to others, share and learn from them. Share your experiences with them, too. We have to believe in ourselves and our ability to live well. If we do, and if we have the determination and perseverance to achieve our personal goals, anything is possible.

For more information, contact Marie at fit4ms@hotmail.com.

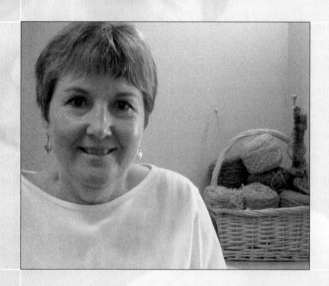

CHAPTER 12

The Knotty Knitters

LOIA FEUCHTER

AFTER MY DIAGNOSIS, I taught school for another twenty-three years. When the MS finally slowed me down to the point where I had to retire, I thought about what I might do next. I loved to knit, so I started a knitting guild. At first there were just six of us in my living room, but now we're up to fifty-four members! We do philanthropic knitting, mostly. Lap robes for caring companions, preemie caps for local hospitals, teddy bears for the fire department to hand out to scared kids, scarves for the men on the Mississippi Riverboat, blankets for a local children's cancer ward. I am so proud to have been able to use this age-old art to touch hundreds of lives. Without my MS, none of this would have happened. ——————————————————————

When I'd been married just two years I was told I had a demyelinating disease, a deteriorating of the myelin sheath around the nerves. The doctors told me I would need a spinal tap for a more precise diagnosis, but since my only symptom was a tingling sensation when I bent my neck down, I decided to just ignore it. Six years later, in 1978, I was diagnosed with optic neuritis in my left eye. I couldn't see for ten days. That was the first time the doctors said the words "multiple sclerosis." Up until that time they had just kind of skirted the issue. But hearing those words it hit me, "Wow, this is it. I'm going to be confined to a wheelchair for the rest of my life."

I didn't let the thought last long. I did some research and discovered that not everyone with MS ends up in a wheelchair and that there are lots of ways to work around this disease. In fact, after my sight returned I went right back to work and continued teaching fourth, fifth, and sixth graders for twenty-three years!

But it was the MS that finally caused me to retire. I was just so tired. I had to get up at 5 A.M. to get out of the house by 7:30 A.M. to get to school. Then I would work my day. School was over at 3 P.M., but it would take until 4:30 P.M. to get myself together to leave. It was taking every ounce of my energy and I had nothing left for my family. School, home, and sleep. That was my life.

One day my neurologist said, "You know, Loia, there are other things in life besides teaching." I hadn't even considered quitting as an option, but we talked about it and, yes, it was going to be financially, uh, not such a good thing, but I just decided that having quality time with my family was worth it. So I retired. Suddenly I had nothing *but* time on my hands. Okay, I thought, now what? I'm not going to sit around here and feel sorry for myself, but what can I do with myself?

I may not have had school bells and alarm clocks to answer to, but teaching was still in my veins. Thinking about what I could teach, I realized that knitting was a skill I would love to share. So that's when I started the Knotty Knitters. At first there were just six of us. We would get together at my house—my mother, my sisters, my friend Sandy, my aunt, and me. My aunt was a longtime knitter and she brought over all her *Cast On* magazines—the national magazine for the Knitting Guild of America—along with a trunk filled with her gorgeous hand-made sweaters. Browsing through the magazines one day, we stumbled on an article about an upcoming conference for knitting guilds in Santa Cruz, California.

I said, "Hey, guys, wouldn't it be fun to check out this conference?" So we flew up to Santa Cruz and met all these wonderful knitters and learned about their guilds and how to form our own guild. We started ours before we even left the conference. I offered to be president because I knew I could organize the guild and I had an idea of how I wanted it to go and what I wanted it to be. My sister then offered to be the secretary because, as she said, "I like to take notes." Sandy chimed in, "I'll be the treasurer because you know I like to take care of money." We decided then and there that our dues would be five dollars.

When we came back from Santa Cruz, I sent off all the paperwork, then ran a little ad in our local paper that read, "Knitting is not a solitary hobby. Come join the Knotty Knitters." I listed my home address and invited anyone interested to join us the first Saturday of every month. That first Saturday twelve knitters showed up. They became the first twelve members of the Knotty Knitters. We decided on our first three goals:

- to learn new things about knitting
- to share what we knew
- to improve our skills

But we all wanted to do something philanthropic, too, so I passed out booklets I had purchased for that first meeting to give the ladies patterns and ideas about the kind of knitting we could do for others. That's when we decided our fourth goal: to knit for others.

We agreed that our first philanthropy project would be to knit preemie caps for the St. Jude's Hospital in Fullerton. That was back in 1995.

Today we have fifty-four members and we've knitted hundreds of preemie caps for St. Jude's and others. When we outgrew my house, I called a church to see if we could use some of their space. The receptionist asked me what we did that had to do with the church? I told her that we knit lap robes for Caring Companions, preemie caps, hats for stuffed bears—Precious Pals—for the fire department. Before I finished rattling off all the projects, we had a new meeting place.

We don't ever force anyone to do philanthropy knitting. Members know that if they want to do it, patterns are available. But once a member knits her first preemie cap or teddy bear sweater, she keeps going. I remember when we first started there was a member who said she only knitted for her family. But as she watched the others making the adorable preemie caps, she said, "Well, maybe I could do a preemie cap, but only one." Well now she's knitting sweaters for the bears and she just finished a lap robe. Knitting for those in need is kind of catching.

Our philanthropy work keeps us busy. We knit bright-colored scarves for the Seamen's Institute in New York for the men on the Mississippi Riverboat. We knit blankets for Project Linus, which we supply to the Loma Linda Children's hospital cancer ward. Then we have a pattern that's called a Five-Hour Baby Sweater, which grew out of a project directed at families trying to break patterns of child abuse.

Then, of course, there are the Precious Pals—the stuffed teddy bears—we do for the Knitting Guild of America. Our ladies just go crazy with design— hippopotamus sweaters and giraffe vests and more. We give these pals to local fire and police departments and they take them on their runs. When they come across traumatized children, they give them a dressed teddy bear. One time the fire company brought their truck right to our meeting so we could load it with bears! We've knitted for the Fullerton Fire, Fullerton Police, Anaheim Fire, Anaheim Police, Garden Grove Fire, and Garden Grove Police, and now we're giving to the Santa Ana Police, too.

It was so gratifying to know that I had started this and had increased awareness of MS at the same time, but at some point I had the itch to see this thing grow. So I applied for, and won, a grant from a company that manufactures a treatment for multiple sclerosis.

I invited seventy people throughout the Southern California Knitting Guild to an "MS Knit-In." My neurologist spoke and presented a slide presentation about MS and followed with a question and answer session. Then, I passed around tote bags with yarn and patterns that I had bought with the money from the grant. Each bag had enough yarn for five philanthropic projects. I described each project and explained which yarns were to be used for each, and then instructed the knitters to return in two months with their finished projects. "We'll have the Return of the MS Knit-In! You'll bring your finished project, a representative from each of the philanthropies will be here to collect them, and then we will have another neurologist speak on the latest MS research."

At the "Return," we had sweaters for the Children's Bureau, lap robes for Caring Companions, scarves and caps for the Seamen's Institute, preemie caps, and lots of teddy bears dressed in new sweaters. You could feel the excitement. I knew I had accomplished both of my goals—to knit for the philanthropies and to educate about MS—when one lady said, "[You have] so much knowledge to give—not just knit one, pearl two, cast on, bind off . . . but relapsing, remitting, secondary progressive, primary progressive, and ABCR Drugs."

Every member of the local guild knows that without my MS, the guild would not have been founded. The obstacles I have overcome have made others aware of MS and the need for more research to develop a cure. I am so proud to have been able to direct my positive attitude toward an age-old art that is touching hundreds of lives.

Anyone interested in forming a knitting guild can visit *www.tkga.com*.

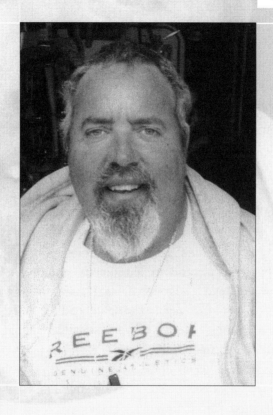

CHAPTER 13

I Wasn't About to Just Stop Living

MARK BLUM

I'M JUST A REGULAR GUY doing something for others. Everybody has something to give, within themselves, something they can share. _____

I've got the worst form of MS, chronic progressive. I was diagnosed in 1993 and worked until March of 1994 in my job as vice president of an insurance company. At that point I couldn't handle the daily routine of work because of the fatigue. But I was forty-two years old and needed something to do. I had a very strong work ethic and wasn't about to just stop living. I had worked on bikes as a child, so I decided to try a bit of bike repair. I certainly had the time.

I found a few adult three-wheelers to work on and found that I really enjoyed it. So, sitting there in my garage, tinkering with the bikes, I came up with the idea for Mission With Bikes. I'd get people to donate broken bikes, fix them up, and give them away for free. I converted my garage into a bike shop and the idea just took off from there.

I fixed the first seventy-five or eighty bikes myself, but because of the MS I lost manual dexterity, and I became legally blind due to nystagmus. But I didn't let this stop me. I began to teach bike repair on a volunteer basis to the local school district. While I can't do that anymore, at the time it kept my mission alive.

Almost ten years later Mission With Bikes is still going strong. So far we've given away 1,447 bikes—all for free. I open up around 6 A.M. and don't close until after 9 P.M., seven days a week. All the bikes are fixed by volunteers. I've got people coming from all over Southern California to work on the bikes. A guy in the Jay Leno Band even comes to help. I've also received many donations of bikes; right now I have about 250 piled up on the side of my house ready to be fixed and given away. The only thing we don't do here is paint them because I don't want that kind of facility in my garage.

I've had volunteers from the Scouts, the Big Brothers, and the police. I've even had the captain of the sheriffs working on bikes in my garage. He helped us last June when we gave thirty bikes to a very poor, inner-city school. The bikes were given out as rewards for perfect attendance to fifteen boys and fifteen girls. I was sent their sizes and ages, and we sent a bike to each child. But this year we hope to have a lot more kids because when they got their bikes the kids were overheard saying, "I'm going to get a bike even if I gotta go to school every day."

I gave one bike to a little girl from Russia who had been brought to the United States for medical treatment. She took that one back to Russia with her. I've given sixty bikes to the Navaho and Hopi Indians. That was quite an experience. An eighteen-wheeler owned by the Airforce National Guard pulled up to my house and four guys in fatigues just jumped out, loaded them up, thanked me, and drove off. Part of my mission is to get bikes to kids who don't have the money to buy them. I occasionally get letters from the kids, which is really rewarding. One time I got a letter of thanks from a kid who explained that when he was five years old his father promised to get him a bike, but he was murdered. Now he finally had a bike.

I've given well over 300 bikes to the homeless in this valley as well as Feme Valley through Lutheran Social Service. Having the bikes makes it possible for them to go to job interviews and get the services they need.

I have raffle bikes and give-away bikes. Of course I never sell them, so I work very well with the local bike shop—Newbury Park Bicycle Shop—which gives me a big price break on parts. They also refer people to me who have bicycles they want to donate.

I've given away 310 individual bikes, including one to a ninety-one-year-old man! What a great feeling to watch that man climb on the bike and take off riding.

I was sitting here in the garage about a year ago when the phone rang. I answered it and some guy said he had read an article about me in a magazine and wanted to donate a case of bike lubricant. I said, "Oh that's great, thank you very much," and we talked for a few minutes. At the end of the conversation I asked where he was calling from and he said Michigan! I've gotten donated parts from Jacksonville, Florida; helmets from all sorts of individuals and churches; tools and other needed items from the Thousand Oaks Do It Center; large trash bins from G. I. Industries; approximately $20,000 worth of bicycle parts from Klockers Bicycle Shop in Bell, California; and the list goes on.

Having MS has been a life-changing experience for me. I feel so blessed to have such good people around me. We take care of each other, and that's what life is all about. I wasn't always a very open person, but now I tell anyone who wants to listen that my garage is an open door. It's a wonderful thing. I started Mission With Bikes for selfish reasons—because I needed a job—but it has turned out to be so much more than that. It's my life.

To donate a bike, parts, or volunteer contact Mark at 818-991-5805.

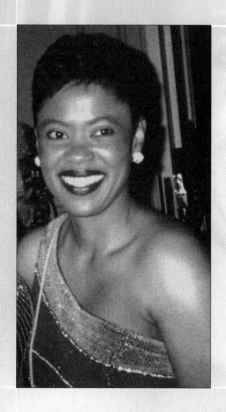

CHAPTER 14

Discover Your Gifts and Share Them

PAM ALLEN

I MAY NEVER AGAIN BE ABLE to play softball competitively, or run a 10K in under fifty minutes, or pack two days' worth of activities and tasks into one day, but that's not important to me anymore. I have learned that I can still lead a happy and productive life with MS. _____

In high school I was a "wanna-be" jock. I played softball, ran track, and played powder-puff football. I tried out for basketball but didn't make the team. Honestly, I never played any sport very well, but if love for the sport could compensate for ability, I would have been a pro!

I continued to run and play softball on into adulthood—until that fateful summer day when I was diagnosed with multiple sclerosis.

MS introduced itself to me with numbness and tingling in my hands. I immediately went to see my internist. He could not find any reason for the loss of sensation, so he referred me to a neurologist. My EMG nerve conduction test came back abnormal. The neurologist did not order additional tests, but on the basis of the one unexplained abnormal EMG concluded that I must have carpal tunnel syndrome. He then referred me to a hand specialist. The hand specialist did not perform any tests, but concurred with the neurologist. I was skeptical about the diagnosis because my understanding of carpal tunnel syndrome was that it was painful and I wasn't experiencing any pain in my hands. But, not having another explanation of what was causing my hands to feel numb and tingly, I accepted the diagnosis. I spent the next two years in and out of hand braces to treat the supposed carpal tunnel.

The second clue that the diagnosis of carpal tunnel syndrome was not correct came in 1994 when I was on vacation with my family. My husband and I had just learned to scuba dive and we were on our first dive trip. We had just finished diving and as we were taking our gear back to our van I noticed that my legs were beginning to get that same numb and tingly sensation. I knew that carpal tunnel syndrome could not account for this, so I went back to my internist. He then referred me to a second neurologist, who narrowed the problem to three possibilities: a tumor on my brain, a tumor on my spine, or multiple sclerosis. I didn't even know what multiple sclerosis was! I figured I had a tumor and was sure they would find it and remove it and life would go on. But when my new neurologist ordered additional tests, including MRIs (with and without contrast), and a lumbar puncture, the results pointed pretty strongly toward MS.

I was devastated. The neurologist's office assistant gave me some literature on MS and suggested that I call the National Multiple Sclerosis Society for more. I followed her advice. I was determined to learn as much as I could about this disease that had invaded my body.

My neurologist had also suggested that I adjust my responsibilities and activities so that I wouldn't get too fatigued or overheated. At the time I had two young children, a full-time job, a husband, and a household to maintain. I couldn't possibly adjust my responsibilities or activities! I was sure that my life as I had known and enjoyed it was over. I was so afraid of not being able to fulfill all of my responsibilities. I sank into one of the darkest emotional places I have ever been.

While I was in this state of darkness, which was actually denial and depression, my oldest daughter reached the age where she could play T-ball. Halfway through the T-ball season, her team's coach had to quit because of changes in his work schedule. A few of the other parents knew of my love and past experience with softball and asked me if I would take over. Without even considering it I said no, but I didn't want to tell them why. At that point I hadn't told anyone outside of close friends and family that I had MS. They kept asking and asking, and I kept saying no!

Finally one of the parents begged me to do it just "until they found someone to take over," and I figured that was something I could do. Of course they never found a coach, and with help from my husband, I ended up finishing the season.

That turned out to be one of the best things that could've happened to me. For the first time in over a year I was not focused on myself and the disease. I found myself looking forward to practice, and I just loved teaching the kids the sport that I had loved for so many years. I learned so much that summer and felt like I had been given a fresh start at life! I learned that if I focused on helping others, and not on myself and the disease, my life could still be as fun and exciting as it had been before MS. That was a life-changing revelation.

I may never again be able to play softball competitively, or run a 10K in under fifty minutes, or pack two days' worth of activities and tasks into one day, but that's not important to me anymore. I have learned that I can still lead a happy, fulfilling, and productive life with MS. I still assist with my daughter's softball team, giving the girls pointers on batting, fielding, or hitting. I also keep score during the games. I also have friends and family members who run many of the local road races, and whenever possible I am there to cheer them on.

I have become more organized in the rest of my life, too. I prioritize my tasks and activities and realize that anything I don't get to do today can wait until tomorrow.

I have also had the opportunity to speak to people from all over the country who have MS. I try to encourage them to take charge of their lives so that they aren't in the darkness of depression and denial. We all have talents and interests that others can benefit from. Although sometimes it's tough, we cannot let MS strip us of our identities. By continuing to pursue our interests and share our talents with others, we will lead happier, healthier, and more fulfilling lives. All it takes is the Courage to Give!

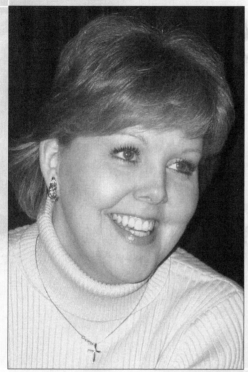

CHAPTER 15

Anne Berry, Trevelyan Studios

Taking the Path God Chose for Me

HOLLY WOODARD

I COULD NEVER HAVE PLANNED or pictured my life turning out this way. I had no specific interest or knowledge in health care or medical equipment. But my diagnosis changed my outlook on everything. I began to understand the importance of insurance and what a lack of it can mean. By providing medical equipment and building ramps for people who can't afford it and helping people get online, I feel more empowered, more capable of helping others see the possibilities of living with a disability. _____

It was the spring of 1996. For three months, I had been experiencing numbness, heaviness, and tingling in both my legs, and for a couple of weeks floppiness in my right foot. I went to my chiropractor because I thought I had a pinched nerve. He tried various tests and referred me to a neurosurgeon. The neurosurgeon ordered an MRI on my brain. He then referred me to a neurologist who ordered MRIs on my upper and lower spine.

In July, my husband and I went in for the results; we had only been married about nine months. When the neurologist told us I had MS, I was actually relieved.

I had been told it might be Parkinson's disease. I knew nothing about MS, but I did know something about Parkinson's and thought MS had to be better. My husband was stunned. He really hadn't thought it was anything serious.

By November, the fatigue and inability to walk very far without assistance was seriously impairing my ability to do my job. I was forced to leave the high pressure and fast pace of multifamily real estate and decided to go back to school for a computer degree so I could start a business at home. I didn't know what type of business I would start, but it seemed like the only way to go. I couldn't have made the transition without the information and support I received from my local MS chapter.

About nine months later, I fell and broke my leg. I had to get a walker instead of crutches since I was still in school and had a backpack to carry. The walker cost $160! I couldn't believe that a couple of pieces of bent metal could cost that much. I was lucky; I had insurance to cover it, but I couldn't help but wonder how the elderly and people on a fixed income could possibly afford such equipment. I live in rural North Carolina. Folks around here aren't rich. How many people were going without the equipment that would allow them even the minimum of mobility and freedom?

I talked to friends who worked in health care and equipment fields. They all said the same thing: If you want to help people, start a nonprofit.

So that is what I decided to do. Mind you, this was quite the opposite of the life I had in mind. I would now be an unpaid volunteer doing something of everything to keep a nonprofit afloat.

I incorporated IMAGINE in January 1998, and we received our federal non-profit status later that year. Two good friends with an interest in helping others and a passion for the mission of IMAGINE started out with me. We decided that we would focus on all the people who were falling through the cracks of the state and federal systems, and we would do it on the honor system. Anyone who was a legal resident of North Carolina who asked for help would get it.

That's how it still works today. We do not ask a lot of personal questions about income and insurance. Our "revolving gift" program allows people with disabilities to use our equipment for as long as they need it and then return it when they're through. We then refurbish it and re-gift it. All our equipment comes through donations.

I could never have planned or pictured my life turning out this way. I had no specific interest or knowledge in health care or medical equipment. But my diagnosis changed my outlook on everything. I began to understand the importance of insurance and what a lack of it can mean. By doing this work I feel more empowered, more capable of helping others see the possibilities of living with a disability.

We are currently celebrating our fifth year of service with IMAGINE, and our service has expanded. Through corporate sponsorships we are now able to build modular ramps and give donated computers and Internet service, along with connection to our statewide listserve, to homebound individuals with disabilities.

Last year we began an annual Adopt-A-Ramp Festival and were able to build two ramps—one for a five-year-old named Colin, who has cerebral palsy. He is so sweet and has such a gorgeous smile. He immediately won over all the volunteers! It poured the whole day we were there, but Colin had a blast and created an atmosphere of love and laughter. We finished the ramp and everyone had a great time. The following week we came back to take photos of Colin coming down his ramp with his mother, and he laughed so hard every time. He begged her to take him up and down the ramp again and again. That is what the gift of giving is all about.

Since my diagnosis, I have gotten involved in my community in all kinds of ways. For five years, I have been teaching Sunday school for adults with developmental disabilities; I work with my local MS chapter as a volunteer ambassador; I work with the North Carolina Citizen Advocacy Network (NCCAN) on statewide advocacy on health-related issues; and serve as a peer counselor.

I am blessed to have a wonderfully supportive husband. Because of him, I have two talented and compassionate stepchildren whom I could not love more if they were my own. I have friends and family who support me regardless of whether or not I have MS.

My life has changed dramatically in the last few years—all for the better. MS has brought many blessings into my life, and has given me an outlook that I never even came close to before. All these things are possible because of the path that God chose for me.

For more information: *www.ifuimagine.org*

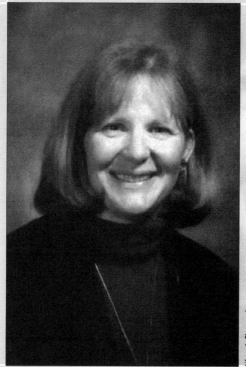

CHAPTER 16

Lifetouch Photographs

You Must Live Your Life Anyway!

CAROLE BISKAR

S OMEONE ONCE SAID THAT living with MS is like living with a terrorist. You never know when it will attack. That is probably true. But you can prepare. Get information, and be proactive about taking care of the symptoms. Find a neurologist you respect and who will take the time to answer your questions. There are many advances in MS treatments—more now than ever before because we know so much more than before. Take small steps or big ones, but realize it is your journey. You may need to get rid of what you have been planning in order to get on with what is waiting for you—or maybe not. Even with MS, be determined to live your life. ⎯⎯⎯⎯⎯⎯⎯⎯⎯⎯⎯⎯⎯⎯⎯⎯⎯⎯

My English grandparents were married for over fifty years when my grandma passed away. It was the first Christmas my grandfather would be alone, so I telephoned him and asked if he would like to come spend it with my family. Fortunately he was able to make the trip. I asked him to tell me about the holiday traditions he and grandma had shared so that I might recreate the kind of Christmas he had shared with her. It seemed like every day he sent names of products and recipes that I'd never heard of. My friends and I were driving all over the Portland area trying to find just the right English toffees, recipes for French onion soup—cooked with just a little sherry—all for Christmas Eve, and ingredients for hot toddies, which I had never made before. I found the steak and kidney pie for Christmas breakfast, the special port wine from England, and I decorated the house with what I had hoped would bring back good memories for him.

All went very well on Christmas Eve. On Christmas morning, my parents and grandpa, my own family, and I sat around a large table looking at these rather unusual steak and kidney pies, the special port wine and various other "delicacies." My father looked up from this breakfast and said, "Dad, I don't remember doing any of this for Christmas. My grandpa held my hand, winked at me, and said, "Oh no, Grandma would have never allowed any of this. This is the way I always *wanted* Christmas to be."

That's what it was like for me with MS. After my diagnosis I needed to redefine who I was and create a new life *with* MS—so that when I look back I will say it was the way I always wanted it to be.

Joseph Campbell, one of my favorite authors, wrote, "We must get rid of what we have been planning so we can get on with what is waiting for us." As synchronicity would have it, I read this right before the telephone call that confirmed my MS diagnosis. I had lost a great deal of vision in my right eye, and after a short run I found most of my right side was numb. It came and went. On morning walks or runs with my husband I had tripped and fallen on a few occasions. We laughed a bit about it, almost nervous laughter, because deep inside we both knew something was wrong. I would close my bad eye when I was working on the computer or writing. But I hid it from people as much as I could.

As a first step, and what I had hoped was my last step, I went to my ophthalmologist for an eye exam. He and his two assistants kept looking at each other, scribbling notes and not really answering me. I knew something was up. At the end of the exam he told me that he couldn't correct the poor vision in my right eye; he ordered one more test and said he would call me. The next morning at work he phoned early and asked to get the name of my family doctor. He told me he would call her and make an appointment for me so I could get in as soon as possible. It was unsettling. I asked him what he thought it might mean. He said, "It could be one of three things: a stroke, a brain tumor, or multiple sclerosis."

I asked, "Do I get a fourth choice?" In his mind, there wasn't one.

My family doctor took me in right away. After asking me a few questions, he encouraged me to see a neurologist—again, right away. The neurologist ordered two MRIs and took my spinal fluid and a case history. His initial thought was that I had MS, and the tests confirmed it.

At that point in my life, I had known only one person with MS. Eighteen years ago, Judy had died rather young of complications related to this disease. I saw myself as being handed a death sentence. I was terrified.

I quilt. I choose my fabrics carefully, the patterns are coordinated, but MS added a new fabric to my quilt, one that I hadn't chosen, and initially it didn't look like it belonged. My design had changed. My journey began. I was now on a very different path than the one I had planned, but heeding Joseph Campbell's words, I spent time trying to accept and understand what was waiting for me. How would I deal with this? I didn't really know—there was no manual, no instructions, no way to get an A on this assignment.

What I did know was that when I was diagnosed with MS the diagram of who I was immediately changed. I am a wife, mother, daughter, redhead, quilter, traveler, friend, adjunct college professor, elementary principal, writer, runner, dog lover, but suddenly MS became the dominant feature of my identity. It really overshadowed everything else. I knew I basically had a choice: I could be a happy person with MS or an unhappy person with MS. I didn't want to live a life of fear and doubt. I believe that fear and doubt stop many of us from fully being what we are capable of. They don't leave much room for joy, compassion, hope, or personal growth. And that was what I wanted—to be genuinely happy and contribute to my family and work.

To start, I wrote down everything that I needed to do to erase my fear and doubt. I learned as much as I could about the disease. I visited MS chat lines and the FDA Website, checked out library books, and sent for pamphlets. I became friends with a woman who also had MS. She was positive and helpful and became a role model for me. My MS circle grew smaller. I learned to accept support and encouragement from others and to ask for help, which was hard at first.

As the information increased, the fear lessened. I had an excellent neurologist who helped me make some decisions. I learned about the ABCR treatments, chose the suggested treatment, and began injecting immediately. Staying healthy also meant getting rest—I need a good eight hours, and my exercise now includes more stretches. MS is now a part of my life, but not *all* of it. It is just one more checkmark on the list of who I am.

In the beginning, the journey was anything but easy. It took a while to realize that the real suffering came from always wishing I didn't have MS. I was scared, sad, and depressed. Up to this point, I had always defined myself by what I accomplished. People looked to me to have answers, to be competent, and to know what I was doing. And I was very afraid—afraid that if I couldn't handle this, maybe I was a fake and wasn't really very good at handling anything. People came to me for support—would they quit coming? Folks asked me for help. Would they stop asking? My parents had always been able to count on me, and now I would worry them. I was liked and loved in part because I was competent and fun to be with. Would people quit liking and loving me? My son looked at me with admiration—would it change to pity?

This disease knocked me off my feet. At a particularly low point I visited my minister, not really sure what I wanted to talk about. I told him of my fears of simply not being good enough any longer and that I was even more afraid of allowing others to see my fear. Sometimes I would park my car on the side of the road and just start crying. I kept makeup in my car so no one would know. I didn't recognize the fears, or even label them.

I also told my minister all of the things I was going to do to "beat this thing." I shared my strategies for my attack. I wanted to be the best MS patient. I told him I wanted to be like the gal on *Oprah*, you know, the woman who has had a hard time, horrible obstacles, and everyone says that she still continued on. No one saw her cry; she never complained, lost a day of work, etc., etc. I want to be that perfect person with this disease. I wanted the A.

He looked at me and said, "Carole, you do not need to be the poster child for MS. You do not need to be or do anything else than what Carole can do. What you have inside is enough—it is more than enough, it is all you need." And finally I breathed a sigh of relief. What he said resonated with me.

There is no magic formula. It looks a little different with each person. I began to look inside for support as diligently as I had looked outside. I realized that I had started to doubt myself, and his words reminded me of my own strength. I had forgotten that. Or maybe I never really understood it in the first place.

Business consultant and author William Bridges writes about changes and transition. He believes, and I agree, that we can't have successful beginnings without good endings. I couldn't begin this life with MS until I began the difficult process of saying goodbye to some things that were me.

The surprise came when I realized that some of the changes felt even better.

I realized, for instance, that since my diagnosis I had had experiences that I simply wouldn't have had before MS. I have had the opportunity to feel a great deal of human kindness, understanding, and compassion, but not pity. Some days I may only garden for forty-five minutes instead of five hours, but it's different now. I enjoy every tiny minute. A parent, one of my PTA officers, came into my office one day and told me that I was her inspiration, because I was always happy, brave, and getting things done at school. I was still enjoying the children and planning things for the school. I appreciated that so much more now than I would have *before.*

But I also told her that I do cry sometimes, that I have my hard days and days when it isn't easy and I don't have courage. I also told her that everyone has some kind of demon at some time in their life, and we all struggle. I suddenly realized that I didn't *want* to be that woman on *Oprah.* That would have been a lie for me. I wanted her to know that. All of a sudden, being perfect didn't seem that important. Being genuine was.

There have been paradoxes with MS. I've slowed down, but I see more. I am not as hard on myself. When I get tired, I rest. Once recently I needed to cut a shopping trip short with my sixteen-year-old son after we had been to only three stores. He put his arm around me, gave me a kiss and said, "Mom, I hate to say it, but there are some good things about you having MS. I didn't want to spend all day here. That's what *you* usually do." He held my hand all the way to the car, not saying anything else.

Shortly after my diagnosis a teacher came by my office and said, "In our new school we will make sure the door is large enough in case you ever need a wheelchair. You will always be our principal." I was so afraid they wouldn't want me with this disease. Their vote of confidence was overwhelming.

I have learned that some days I may need to change plans. When I invite friends for dinner I let them know they might get a nice Brazilian dinner or maybe pizza, depending on how I am doing. And people understand. My husband's roles have changed, too. When I was first diagnosed he said, "Carole, it is no problem. I am here. I will *always* carry you." And he has, in so many ways. He has only had one request of me—to keep my sense of humor—and I've tried.

Sometimes someone with MS will come to my office who, for whatever reason, has been keeping it very private. It is nice to know they want to talk with me. Maybe I am still serving people, but in a different way. I'd like to think so. I have made small day-to-day changes. These days I use a number system with people closest to me, a kind of code that saves a lot of talk about my health. When they ask me how I am, I give them a number from 1 to 10. If I say 1, my secretaries screen my calls and step in a little more than usual. I actually think I'm a much better principal now; I can't chair so many committees, so my staff has stepped forward. We are forging a model of shared leadership, which is the culture I always wanted to create.

This disease isn't easy. It doesn't play fair; it is a change, and it's hard to understand. There is never a day that I *want* to have MS. But I am continuing to do the things I love, with the people I love. I am looking forward to so many things in life. The present seems so much sweeter. My last MRI showed one less lesion, and another is considerably smaller than it was a year ago. Is it because I'm using one of the ABCR treatments? I don't know for certain. But my experience certainly supports the research that I had read in the beginning—that getting on treatment early can make a difference.

I have a drinking glass with a white line painted exactly around the middle. Above the white line is the word *optimisto,* below the white line is written *pessimisto.* My wish for you is that your cup is always filled above the white line. There are more reasons to be optimistic about MS treatment and what we know about the disease than ever before.

My grandpa chose to redesign his Christmas. Remember, you have choices, too.

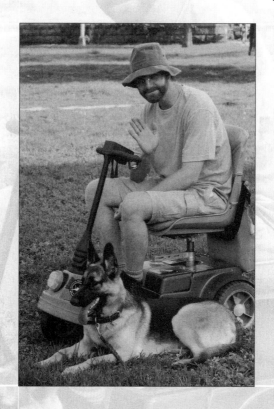

CHAPTER 17

*The Healing Spirit of Faith,
Creativity, and Companionship*

DR. BRETT WEBER

THE WEEK BEFORE COMPLETING my Ph.D. in neuroscience at Temple University, I was diagnosed with primary progressive multiple sclerosis (MS). I have partial paralysis in my left leg, have difficulty standing, and must use a wheelchair. As a scientist, I had focused on how the brain processes visual information. I also studied nerve regeneration. Since my diagnosis, I have devoted myself to understanding this disease through scientific research, but also through my art.

Of course MS can be devastating to those who are afflicted with it and to their families, but like any major life-changing event chronic illness can also bring new values, new appreciations, and new colors and textures into one's life. It is my hope that through my art I can encourage broader research on MS. _____

I have always admired Leonardo da Vinci. He experimented in both art and science and experienced his share of both success and failure. I admire that attitude to be unafraid, to pursue truth, to have faith in your observations, and to continue onward no matter what obstacles present themselves. In that way, I have always hoped to emulate Leonardo. Not only by doing both art and science, but by pursuing each without fear in an effort to do some good.

There is a sharp distinction between art and science, and studying a disease through art is not the same as studying it through science. My art is about my own emotional, intellectual, and spiritual journey, and within that context MS plays a significant role. When I paint, I feel as though I am on a journey of discovery. I allow myself to think about problems in a different way. As I navigate my own course through an expression of color and texture, I hear the words of great people and imagine the journeys they have taken.

My paintings tell me about my journeys. They are a record of where I have been. Dissimilar as we may be, both artists and scientists are creatures of observation. What some overlook, we take joy in discovering. Things perhaps not clearly understood, but things we believe to be real and open to interpretation. We are in constant struggle to describe what we observe. And even after we convince ourselves and others that we have seen some truth and made sense of it, there is always some doubt. The artist and scientist both recognize how imperfect our human capacity is as we search for moments of understanding in a sea of complexity.

Physicians claim that about one half of all people who have MS experience a serious depression during their illness. I have, of course, at times felt depressed about my situation. Interestingly though, I have never felt compelled to go on any form of antidepressant medication. I believe that I am blessed with a naturally happy disposition but that I have also maximized my natural coping skills through thinking productive positive. For example, how people affect me emotionally has become an important consideration. I simply refuse to be surrounded by negative people—and this includes certain individuals within the medical community. I choose my physicians and my friends very carefully. They have a powerful impact on the way we feel about ourselves—rousing courage and hope, or fear and depression.

A wide range of physical symptoms can come and go over time with MS. The disease causes damage within the central nervous system along nerve pathways affecting movement, speech, vision, hearing, and bladder and bowel control. What is not commonly recognized is that the disease can also directly interfere with a person's ability to think clearly. Damage within the brain can create changes that affect problem solving, attention, learning, and memory. I believe that just as physical therapy can help people with MS maintain as much physical ability as possible, mental therapies that encourage problem solving, attention, learning, and memory skills may help people with MS maintain as much cognitive ability as possible. Strategies such as art therapy and other positive, challenging, creative outlets may help improve or maintain partially impaired cognitive pathways within the brain and may enhance an individual's self-worth and natural coping skills against depression and perhaps fatigue.

A diagnosis of MS implies a lifelong condition, progressive physical disability, emotional conflict, and lasting adjustments. It's not uncommon to experience a sense of disbelief, anger, depression, guilt, fear, and a driving desire to regain control over one's life. All of these negative feelings contribute to an intense and active stress. Stress is a normal reaction to MS and should be expected. But instead of allowing our stress to cripple us further, it can be extremely helpful to find positive stress-relieving escapes from the disease. My escape is my art. My artwork is about bringing unity to myself. It is about listening to instead of shouting at reality. It is also about triggering my mind's unconscious thought processes toward healing—by paying attention to and making sense of the normally silent, repressed, and oftentimes distant elements within myself.

Several years ago a friend of mine referred to a painting that I had just finished as being "either a complete abstraction or a landscape, but either way poetry." That friend convinced me to exhibit my artwork professionally, if for no other reason than to raise public support and awareness for MS and my rare form of the disease.

My paintings are abstractions. I do not intend to paint representational images. From time to time they may appear to be something recognizable, but I never intend to paint anything representational. I do name my paintings (other artists often leave their abstract art untitled), however, and I believe that in searching for a name I usually come to recognize what my paintings represent.

The entire process of creating and then naming my paintings provides me with a very satisfying physical, emotional, intellectual, and spiritual release. What's more, because I approach my artwork with no expectations of good or bad, right or wrong, correct or incorrect, much as a young child first approaches art, I experience very little of the stress and anxiety that is often associated with the creative process. What will people think of my creative work? In view of my illness, questions that used to cause me anxiety (my Ph.D. defense, for example), have become much less important. I create artwork for my own enjoyment now, and to my own personal satisfaction.

For instance, I have come to understand the idea behind my painting *Rainforest* as the act of global deforestation—the cutting, burning, and irretrievable extinction of our planet's most valuable resource: biological diversity. We are losing at an unprecedented pace plant, insect, and animal species that might hold the cures for diseases like MS.

As a scientist who has a disease with no cure, this issue is especially close to me. I see the deforestation of the world's rainforests (and loss of biological diversity) as the single most important issue of our time, and I feel symbolically linked to global deforestation and the burning rainforests with every passing day through the demyelination of nerve cells that is continuing unabated within my own body—someone should listen.

Since September 11, 2001, and my debut as an artist in New York City that December, I have come to see myself as a hostage and my MS as a terrorist—a foreign aggressor within my body whose intent is to inflict great suffering on me and my loved ones through random, ongoing, unstoppable acts of unprovoked violence. But this terrorist has no other cause, and it is non-negotiable.

Recently my dear aunt Shirley sent me a novel called *Bel Canto*. In it Ann Patchett writes, "What begins as a panicked, life-threatening scenario slowly evolves into something quite different, a moment of great beauty, as terrorists and hostages forge unexpected bonds and people from different continents become compatriots. Friendship, compassion, and a chance for great love lead the characters to forget the real danger that has been set in motion . . . and cannot be stopped."

Patchett's description captures the emotional sentiment that I have experienced toward my enemy (MS) as well as my friends. Serving people who are also held hostage by MS (or some other illness) and allowing them to help me has gradually come from my appreciation that although my encounter with my enemy has certainly not been positive, it has also not been entirely negative either. The courage to form bonds in creative expression, spirituality, and/or simply companionship is seeing the love, courage, and beauty that ultimately come to pass during a devastating event—such as the devastation that touched the world on September 11, 2001, and the *Columbia* shuttle disaster on February 1, 2003.

There is a healing spirit that arises within people during times of disaster, when strangers who may momentarily panic, flee, or fall into despair grow closer as companions, find their common faith, and act with creative boldness. So it has been with my illness, friends, and family.

This holiday season a friend of mine was asked by her seven-year-old disabled son Aron, "Mom, tell me the truth, why am I in a wheelchair? Why am I the one who has to be in a chair and not walk?" She explained to him "I told you the truth, you have cerebral palsy (CP) and that part of your body was the most affected." He nodded, "I know that part, but tell me the truth. Why is it me?"

When she asked what I would say to him, hinting for some creative boldness, I told her I did not know, but shared with her the words that this thirty-two-year-old man repeats to himself everyday: I am a soldier and I am on a mission. My mission is to *not* be afraid, to not be angry. I have those orders from my superior officers, my faith and close companions, who tell me regularly that I have been given all that I need. War is tough! The mission does not seem possible at times, but I am a soldier, and I will not let my commander and my fellow soldiers down who fight alongside of me.

What we all must remember daily is that we are *not* alone, and that we have won many battles together. We can expect to win the war. No doubt! No fear.

It is true that some people live easier lives than we do. And some live more difficult lives. We must be soldiers. Not everyone is a soldier. And not everyone sees the enemy. But we see the enemy, we have our orders, and we must *not* be afraid.

I have never actually been a soldier, but I understand the mission of fighting for a cause, not one that you have chosen but one that has chosen you.

At our former home near Philadelphia we lived close to a pavilion where one afternoon a group of veterans who had fought in various wars were enjoying some music and a violent summertime storm after placing some 58,168 small American flags side by side in a soccer field, commemorating each person who died in the Vietnam War (and a smaller circle of flowers remembering the victims of September 11, 2001).

I only intruded because I was on my scooter without an umbrella in a downpour. When I arrived under the pavilion, soaking wet, with my German shepherd service dog, Sophia, I was immediately offered a cigarette and a towel. I dried off and shared some banter about the lightning flashes and my dog. Jimi Hendrix music was blaring, and a wickedly powerful thunderbolt came down before it dawned on me that everyone under the pavilion thought I was just another veteran. They talked to me as though I had known them my entire life. It was a good feeling, and I was relieved that no one asked me how I came to be in a scooter or what war I served in. At the time I felt that my answer of MS would have disappointed them, but now I think otherwise. These guys understood war and irony, but those were topics for some other time. This day was about companionship and planting flags in the ground during a marvelous summer storm.

Leonardo da Vinci once referred to art as being "the queen of all sciences"— a queen who offers not simply an alternative approach to obtaining knowledge but also a way of sharing that knowledge with the world. Although MS has affected my hands to some degree, I choose to do abstract art not because of my reduced dexterity but because abstraction is the only style of art that can be executed without planned intent, and is therefore a way for me to dream.

Through my art I wish to issue this warning: As fellow passengers on planet Earth, we must recognize our common natural enemy as disease. Never has there been an enemy who has touched more people, and there will never be an enemy who will take more lives. Since the dawn of human civilization we have waged war against this enemy through our shamans, witchdoctors, and now scientists. Our scientists must be our frontline soldiers, and they must wage a different kind of war for us in this new millennium. Not a war against neighbors who may define art, science, or God as being something different from our own immediate and limited understanding. No. Let us make peace with our brothers and sisters and fight the one Holy War on Earth—the war against human illness.

For additional information visit *www.brokenartgallery.com*

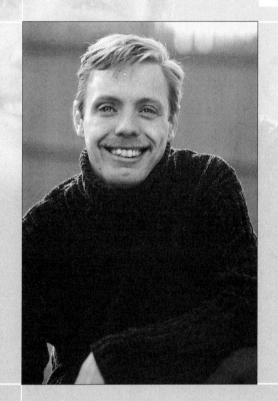

CHAPTER 18

A Box to Put My MS In

MATT OELFKE

D EALING WITH MS is a lifelong challenge, and I refuse to succumb. I want people to know that MS is only a single part of our lives, one that we cannot allow to rule our lives. We all have to remember one thing: we have MS but MS does not have us. _____

Being diagnosed with MS is hard to deal with at any age, but at age twenty-five my diagnosis was especially difficult for me. I had recently injured my back from a ten-foot fall at my construction job. Eighteen months later, my back problems, along with emerging MS symptoms including double vision, body pain, diffi- culties in controlling my bladder and walking, and numbness, kept me from working altogether. This made my wife, who was at the time pregnant with our first child, the sole financial supporter of the family.

I felt so helpless, I was just ready to give up. Here I had gone from working in a profession that relies on strength and stamina to living with a disease that left me barely able to walk. But I began to think about my unborn child and remembered a promise I had made to myself when I was young: to be a respon- sible father and raise my children well. This was a promise I intended to keep. I simply couldn't let MS control my life.

Like all expecting parents, I started to "baby proof" our home, which meant, among other things, safeguarding all my syringes, needles, alcohol wipes, and medicine for my injections, so they would be out of our newborn's reach. Plus,

I thought it would be better to have these things out of sight; otherwise they would be a constant reminder of my disease.

To store them safely, I built a wooden box with several compartments, including a space to prepare the injections. Then I decided to decorate the box with pictures of my family to make it pleasant to look at as well as functional. Now when I need my supplies, I always get to see a picture of my son, Joey, with his smiling and happy face.

I deliberately designed the box so that it would be as easy as possible to give myself my shots. In the upper part of the box, in the left hand corner, is a space to store used syringes. Next to that is a place for unused syringes, so they're always ready for my next shot. In the lower part of the box, there is space for alcohol swabs and anything else I wish to store there. The front of the box, when it is lowered, provides a tray, which lies flat on a table to prevent anything from rolling off. That way I'm able to take out all the supplies I need and have them right in front of me in one place. When I'm finished giving myself an injection, I can put the used needle in the storage container, close the tray, put the lid down, and I'm done. Having the box gives me both physical and emotional distance from MS. When I leave the box, my MS stays there.

After seeing my box, a fellow MS support group member was so impressed that he asked me to make one for him. Quickly, news about the box began to spread, and a local newspaper reporter asked me for an interview. After the story appeared, I received $6,000 in anonymous donations and numerous little notes of inspiration from MS communities—local and national—asking me to make more boxes.

I could see that making boxes gave me the perfect opportunity to share my experience with other people with MS. Demand has been so great that a manufacturing company now mass produces the boxes. A portion of the proceeds from the sale of each box is donated to MS research. After receiving a grant, I purchased fifty boxes made to distribute to low-income MS patients in my home state of Michigan.

My wife and I are now the proud parents of two children, Joey and Casey. I continue to fulfill that childhood goal of being a good father and a loving husband. Because of my disease, however, I've added another goal: to be a source of motivation to others living with MS. The box has given me a chance to meet this objective.

I hope that my boxes—whether used for storage or as a psychological barrier from the disease or both—will be a source of inspiration for other people with MS.

For more information about the MS Box, log onto *www.theMSbox.com.*

_____

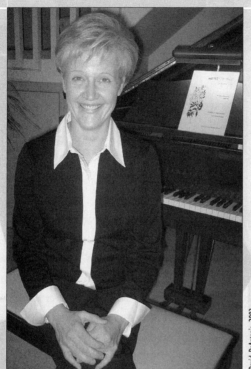

CHAPTER 19

David DeAntonis, 2003

The Universe Always Guides Us in the Right Direction

NANCY HEINE

E VERY TIME I LET MY PASSION lead me and let go of fear, amazing things come my way. With MS, I have been given the gift of seeing just how strong we really are when we find our passion and follow it, no matter what our obstacles may be. _____

My alarm clock went off at 5:00 A.M., as always. It was a cold winter day in 1993 and I had a 6:00 A.M. dance/aerobics class to teach, after which I would run over to the campus to teach two keyboard classes before returning home to my piano studio, when my day would really begin. This particular morning, however, I ended up on the floor. My left leg was numb from my toes to my waist. It felt as though massive doses of Novocaine had been shot into my leg. I had never experienced anything like it before. I made my way over to the phone to call a friend who is a doctor. This was the beginning of my journey with MS.

I spent the next several weeks being referred to one doctor after another and ended up with a neurologist and a seven-day hospital stay, having MRIs, spinal taps, and other tests. My family and friends flew in and were there when I was diagnosed with MS. As I heard the diagnosis and took in what it meant, I thought back over the years and remembered the symptoms that I had always attributed to something else—the fatigue that would stop me in my tracks, a couple of odd falls. The name itself frightened me, but what I was most afraid of was never being able to play the piano again. Teaching aerobics was a fun sideline I could easily give up, but playing and teaching piano was my passion in life.

As I shuffled down the hallway in the neurological floor of the hospital, feeling scared and overwhelmed, I happened to glance into another room and saw a man paralyzed from the neck down. I watched his wife and children talking with him and suddenly realized how grateful I was to be walking at all. I also realized that being grateful is much more fulfilling than feeling cheated out of something. I only hoped I would remember this if I lost the use of my hands.

When I returned home, I went straight to my baby grand and played a song. I can still remember hearing my sister and mother quietly crying in the next room. After I settled into living with MS, my life took another unexpected turn. I started composing, and the music flowed out of me as if it had been there waiting all of my life. After hearing some of my compositions my friend Randy, a dancer/choreographer, asked if I would be willing to write the music for a collaborative work he was doing with Jules Feiffer. I had just started composing, so at first I hesitated. But Randy had been diagnosed with AIDS and this was probably going to be his last big project; how could I say no?

Randy and I worked together for a few months, and Jules Feiffer flew in for the opening. It was a success beyond our wildest dreams. Shortly after the premier of the *Feiffer Dances*, Randy died, but in that short time we had together he helped me for a lifetime. I only hope that in some small way I helped make his last days the best they could be. By saying yes to his project despite the obstacles, I took a chance, and taking that chance not only helped others but fulfilled me unlike anything I'd ever done before.

Word got around and I became known as a composer for dance. It wasn't long before I was asked to do the music for a spot in an AIDS benefit concert. My sister choreographed the dance and I composed the music. Working on a concert for people with AIDS took my mind off the obstacles I was facing with MS.

I occasionally walked with a cane and had had trouble with optic neuritis. But my biggest challenge had been and continues to be the incredible fatigue that accompanies MS. But once again, the experience taught me something invaluable: everyone has their own challenges to face in this life, and it takes work to find the courage to face these challenges.

As I worked with the AIDS patients for the concert, I continued to journal as I had done for years, but I also started a gratitude journal. Each day I found things I was grateful for, like being able to get out of bed, watching a sunset at the beach, or riding horses. What I discovered was the more I was grateful for, the more strength I found within.

Shortly afterward my best friend, who lived in Vancouver, Washington, told me of a job opening that intrigued me—a chance to teach at the Vancouver School of Arts and Academics. After interviewing and taking the job, which was part time and also included teaching at an elementary school, I packed up my baby grand and two cats and moved across the country.

The move was not something I had planned, but I just knew I had to take another chance. Since my diagnosis, my life had become richer and fuller, but there was still one area of my life that did not feel complete. I had been single for forty-five years. It was time to welcome a love relationship into my life. So I decided to take a big chance and do something I never thought I would do—I advertised in the personal ads. I got many responses but returned only one call. I met David for coffee and within the first fifteen minutes told him I had MS. I waited for his reaction. He simply acknowledged it and we kept on talking. We have been talking ever since.

David and I have a deep spiritual connection; I know he came into my life because I needed to learn about reaching out and finding a loving relationship despite the obstacles of having MS. Again, I earned another magnificent gift when I let go of my fear surrounding MS.

My next lesson came from my students in Vancouver. We decided to put on an MS benefit concert. Watching the students compose music, choreograph, write poetry, and perform for the concert was one fulfilling moment after another. It energized me, inspired me, and gave me a new respect for our youth. It gave me the courage to continue to compose and teach and help others, despite the overwhelming fatigue of MS.

When the school year ended I took off for a two-week artist-in-residence program in the Rocky Mountain National Park. For two weeks, I lived in an historical cabin, far away from most people, with only a daily visit from a forest ranger on horseback, bringing me my mail. I had applied for the residency because I wanted to live in the elements to foster love, appreciation, and knowledge of nature. Little did I know that my two passions, music and the environment, would merge as I began to compose music based upon the birds' songs that echoed in the mountains. I completed the music book and donated it to the Rocky Mountain National Park. Once again, a new experience stretched me in ways I could not have foreseen. Staying alone in a rustic cabin with no one to talk with but myself gave me time for reflection.

I began to see a pattern emerging in my life. Every time I let my passion lead me and let go of fear, amazing things would come my way. In this experience I was given the gift of seeing just how strong we really are when we find our passion and follow it, no matter what our obstacles may be. I returned to school and the students with renewed energy and additional wisdom. The school year had barely begun when we had to face September 11, 2001.

On September 12, I walked into my Music Special Projects Class and asked my students, "How do you feel and what can we do?" One student said that he had written a song the night before and that he wanted to send it to New York. We listened to the song with its poignant words and haunting melody and cried together. Out of our mourning we decided what would most help us heal. We committed to compose music, write poetry, and create visual artwork reflecting our love and concern for the people of New York and to compile a book of these works to send to New York for the one-year remembrance on 9/11/02. Once again my students' spirit of giving just amazed me. All year they worked hard composing, drawing, writing, designing the cover, and healing.

One day one of the seniors at school asked if we might get some contributions from my elementary school students. Those contributions turned out to be just the final touch we needed for this miraculous book. When some of the kids were interviewed on a local television news program, they said they wanted people in New York to know that people on the other side of the country loved them—a simple truth but one that we all needed to hear over and over again. Our book, *With an Eagle's Tear,* was published and sent to over thirty different places in New York.

I shudder to think of what my life would be like now if I had continued to live out of fear of losing the use of my hands, not being able to play the piano or compose. The disease itself may have many unknowns, but there are one or two things I know for sure about my life with MS. When I reach out with love to help others, I receive love in return, and this heals me. When I am grateful for what I have, the universe opens up and guides me in the right direction. When I face life's obstacles with courage, life never lets me down.

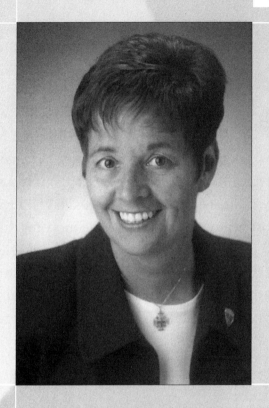

CHAPTER 20

From "I Can't" to "I Can"

SISTER KAREN J. ZIELINSKI

ONE OF THE HARDEST PARTS of living with a chronic illness like MS is thinking that you have to face it alone—but you really don't. Whenever I begin to feel alone, I try to remember to reach out to a friend to help me do errands, pray with me, or just talk. Prayer is probably the most healing thing I do. In the morning, I pour myself a cup of coffee, light a candle, and pray the psalms. I am always struck by the ones that speak of healing. From praying the psalms, my thinking changes from what I can't do with MS to what I can. _____

At first I thought it was my new "industrial strength" support pantyhose that caused the numbness in my legs. It was October of my first year teaching junior high. I went to the doctor, thinking I had pinched a nerve. Three weeks later, I came out of the hospital with a diagnosis of multiple sclerosis. I was twenty-two years old.

That was twenty-eight years ago, and a lot of things have changed for me since then. These days I walk with a cane and wear a leg-strengthening brace.

But for the first twelve years, my MS was mostly dormant—my legs tired easily, but there were no other symptoms. Gradually, the neurological disease progressed, and I decided I had to do something to help me cope. The decision to take control of my MS was not dramatic. It happened over time—and is still happening—through the choices I make.

I think my family background, my faith, and my philosophy of life have made me see the "everybody's got something, nobody's perfect" part of the human condition. Of course, I have moments when I shed tears because I want to do more things, but the fact is, I can't. We humans have many facets: we are physical, emotional, spiritual, sexual, and social beings. For me, the transforming power of MS has come through my spirituality.

I spend a lot of time resting, doing physical therapy, taking medicine, and praying. I'm a Roman Catholic nun with the Sisters of St. Francis of Sylvania, Ohio, and I try to live by St. Francis of Assisi's prayer: "Lord, make me an instrument of Thy peace." I find great comfort in scripture and prayer. Prayer guides me to do things that are right for me. Every time I do my thirty-five-minute mat exercise program in physical therapy, I say a silent prayer. It's the prayer that helps me do these things with hope in my heart.

You know, people have always used prayer, music, ritual imagination, and faith along with traditional therapies to cope with disease. These days we may call these "alternative therapies," but they're such an important part of the healing process. I know that many people in the world of medicine are skeptical of prayer, and I'm grateful that my medical professionals have always supported me in my beliefs.

If I had to pinpoint the major turning points in how I look at this disease, one of them would have to be the night I watched the series finale of *Murphy Brown.* Murphy is just finishing a six-month course of chemotherapy for breast cancer and is at the doctor's office for a final mammogram. She is ready to say to the nurse, "Okay, it's been real, see you in six months," and walk out, but the nurse tells her that the doctor needs to talk with her about a suspicious spot on her breast.

Murphy is scheduled to have exploratory surgery the next day. While under the anesthetic, she has a dream about her job. In her waking life, she's been planning to retire from her job as a top-notch investigative news reporter for a major network news show and enjoy life, because, as she says, "The only person I haven't interviewed is God!" Of course, in her dream, she interviews God.

After a few general questions about God's age, who goes to Heaven, and why evil happens in the world, God answers Murphy's question, "Why in the hell (oops, excuse me, heck) do I have breast cancer?" with the answer, "Your cancer is a gift."

Murphy wakes up to discover that the tumor is benign, goes back to work, and truly experiences a conversion. She is no longer the cynical reporter she once was. Her disease, her gift, transformed her.

Hearing this brought me to tears. I gave myself some time to analyze my feelings and realized that my MS is a gift too.

Of course most people would think this is nuts! I walk slowly with a cane and a leg brace. Everything takes longer, and getting around can be pretty painful. But I have so much to be grateful for. Living with this disease for twenty-three years has shown me just how much love there is in this world. I have so many wonderful people in my life, so many friends who travel with me, shop with me, or go to a movie with me, and support me in my fundraising activities. And then there's Sister Act.

Sister Act is our team for the walk that raises money for the National MS Society's efforts to find a cure. We just celebrated our tenth anniversary. The size of the team changes year to year, but one year we had about twenty sisters walking. We are quite an act. The sisters, who do this as a ministry, range from elementary school principals and teachers, to college professors, to hospital chaplains and physical therapists and nurses. We hope to raise our annual $5,000 this year and bring our grand total to $50,000.

At times I feel that MS is my enemy. But ironically, it has taught me that while life is not perfect, it is still beautiful. It's kind of like a Christmas tree that has a few branches missing; it's still a beautiful tree. My MS has made me see that the human condition is fragile and that people themselves, not what they do, are the most precious gifts of all.

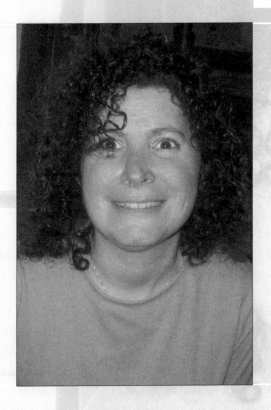

CHAPTER 21

Normalcy Is What You Make It

NICOLE FOULIARD

T HERE IS NOTHING WE CAN'T DO. We might do it a little slower, we might do it a little differently, but we can do it. _____

One morning in 1989, I woke up numb from my mid-thigh to my waist. I didn't think too much about it since it was just a tingling feeling. I have a lot of skin allergies, so I thought that's what it probably was. Except that the numbness was spreading.

A few days later I was really uncomfortable, so I drove to my family's home in Mesa—about a hundred miles away. I was exhausted so I fell asleep on my Mom's couch. When I woke up I was completely paralyzed from the neck down and could only lift my fingertips and my feet. I was so scared. My dad tried to sit me up on the couch, but I was like a rag doll and just slid off.

Miraculously, as fast as the paralysis came, it started going away. Still thinking it was probably just a really bad allergy attack, I decided to head back to school. But about thirty minutes into the drive, I didn't feel safe. Fortunately my grandparents lived between Mesa and Tucson, so I stopped at their house. My grandmother thought it was a pinched nerve in my back. She gave me a muscle relaxant and I went to sleep. Several hours later I woke up feeling much better and drove the rest of the way home.

The next day I went to the medical center at the University of Arizona for an examination. The doctor said I needed to see a neurologist and made a few calls, and within two and a half hours I was in a neurologist's office. Of course, I was freaking out. I figured I had a brain tumor or something.

After an MRI the doctor called and suggested I come in and bring my mother with me. I hung up the phone sure that I was dying.

He sat us down and told us that my symptoms were consistent with multiple sclerosis. I didn't really know what multiple sclerosis was, but of course I started crying. He explained that this was what is called an exacerbation—a bad one that would probably last four to six weeks. He said I would probably get better after that and might even go into remission for fifteen to twenty years but that eventually I would come out of remission and the disease would just slowly progress for the rest of my life. I didn't know any better so I believed him. Thirteen years later I'm still waiting for the remission.

I was a musical theater major at the time, and I remember saying to my mother, "I'm never going to dance again." She laughed and said, "You didn't dance to start with!" At least she made me laugh.

My mom was right; I was a terrible dancer, which makes more sense in hindsight. My terrible sense of rhythm and the fact that I was always breaking bones had to do with my instability, my MS.

During my first year, I lived on and off crutches and in and out of a wheelchair, waiting for the twenty years of remission to set in. I dropped out of college with only a semester until graduation. My mother drove to my house every day to help me with basic needs such as grocery shopping, cleaning, and doctor's visits and to get me out of the house.

Although I had pretty much dropped out of life, I had short periods of normalcy. During one of those periods, I got pregnant, but my partner split. Then by some grace, I did go into remission for a while. Life was good. That's when I realized that no matter how much chaos my life might be in I was the only one who could control my destiny.

My daughter, Alex, was born in June of 1991. When she was sixteen months old, the MS returned with a vengeance. I lost my sight, which was by far the scariest thing that's happened so far, and we had to move back in with my parents. I began to wonder if having a child wasn't a huge mistake.

It took some time, but I began to recognize even the smallest accomplishments as success. I could see color, so I bought Alex all bright colored clothing so I wouldn't lose her while walking her to daycare. My mother made me cook dinner one night a week, so I cooked Mexican food because it has lots of color. I learned to read Braille and listened to books on tape without falling asleep. I learned how to ride buses.

The whole situation was hard on everyone around me, and I knew it. My mother was tired of changing diapers, my twelve-year-old sister was sick of sharing a room with Alex and me, my brother was tired of babysitting. My other sister was sick of having to "help your sister" with even the easiest of tasks, like making sure all the shampoo was out of my hair. My grandmother cried a lot, and my grandfather couldn't even look at me, let alone talk to me.

It took about nine months for everyone to adjust. Then, not even two months later and only when I finally accepted my blindness did my sight start to slowly return! Ah, the beauties of living with a disease with its own agenda.

When I could see well enough to manipulate a computer screen, I returned to school, where I met Paul, my journalism professor. From the start he had nothing but faith in me. He didn't know what baggage I had and he didn't feel sorry for me. He just loved me for who I am. Paul once said that with me he could dream with his eyes open.

Shortly after he proposed, my grandmother was diagnosed with terminal cancer, so we shortened our engagement to six weeks to be sure she'd be there for the wedding. With the stress of my grandmother's illness and a wedding to plan, my sight and mobility started to deteriorate again. In a desperate measure of denial I tried to do extraordinary things. My vision dimming, I not only painted my kitchen table but stenciled it, too. Then I made Alex a quilt by hand. When I look at it today, I see that it's rather awful, but she treasures it and thinks it's great.

On our honeymoon, Paul and I decided another pregnancy would be good for me, so now we have Brett. What luck that was! Brett keeps me mobile and gives me all the exercise I could ever want.

In those days I was so determined to prove that I was still "normal," but now I think I've learned that normalcy is what you make it. Having MS has taught me how to appreciate what I *can* do. It has taught me how to ask for help when I need it and that asking for help doesn't mean I'm inadequate. Having MS has made me pick and choose what I do and to be deliberate in my actions. Some days I can make it up the stairs to kiss Alex and Brett goodnight. Some days, more often than not, they come downstairs to me. But that's not what really matters. After almost thirteen years of battling with and learning how to live with MS, I have learned that having MS does not define who I am.

In 2001, I was named Central New England National MS Society Mother of the Year. Turns out my daughter, Alex, had secretly submitted the application. When I saw what she wrote, I knew that everything I'd been through was worth it.

1. List ways in which this candidate participates in the lives of their children.

Cub Scouts, Girl Scouts, Softball, Hockey, Cheerleading

2. List family activities or hobbies which the candidate participates in with their children

   Plays Nintendo 64 with us, cheers for us at all sporting events, reads books to us, plays board games, and makes up funny stories and jokes when we are not feeling good.

3. Show from candidate's children's point of view, why their parent should be named MS Mother of the Year

   Because she is thoughtful, caring, trusting, loving, and kind and even though she has MS she is the greatest mom ever!

4. Are there any additional facts or stories which you feel are relevant as to why they should be chosen as MS Mother of the Year?

   My mom has been blind, in and out of a wheelchair, on and off crutches and she has always loved me and has never stopped taking care of me.

I never would have believed that thirteen years into my life with MS I would be a wife, the mother of two great kids, a law student, a political activist, and a volunteer in my community. How grateful I am for all of it, but especially for Paul, Alex, and Brett, who believe in me so much and make me dream every day, who make me feel like there is nothing I can't do. I might do it a little slower, I might do it a little differently, but I can do it.

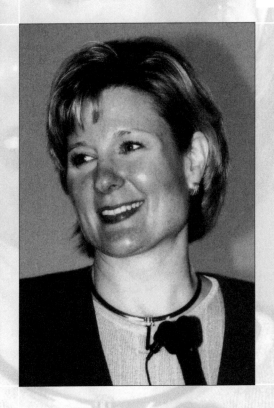

CHAPTER 22

Don't Just Sit There, Do Something

DONNA BOLDT

MS HAS IN SOME WAYS BEEN A BLESSING. It has given me the blessing of establishing new relationships, taking control of my well-being, and sharing my story. _____

For many years my parents and I wondered why I was so forgetful and klutzy. We just assumed it was a way of life. We found out it was more than that. I have multiple sclerosis.

Growing up I was exposed to so many wonderful things. My parents took us all over North America, we skied, boated, hiked, biked; we were exposed to history, art, music. We used to camp in a tent in West Virginia for seven weeks each summer, I got to model with a well-known agency and to participate in various organizations and athletic programs. I was a very, very lucky kid. By the time I reached college I was a pretty good student, a hard worker, and a competing precision sharpshooter. Eventually I climbed to become the third-generation president of our family Chemical Distribution Company—Deeks & Company, Inc.

But although I led an active life, I was always klutzy. I had "mysterious" health problems, even as a small child. I would have bouts of pain in my legs and an inability to walk. My parents took me to every specialist in the state to rule out all of the known diseases. No one could ever tell us what was wrong, but the symptoms would always go away over time. As an adult I became a nationally ranked competitive sharpshooter, so I was obviously steady enough most of the time, but then there were those times when I would knock over my wine glass at dinner, run my sweet husband off the road when we went running, drop things, or fall asleep whenever I sat for more than ten minutes. We'd just laugh and joke about all of my "weird klutzies," and life went on.

But by October of 2000 warning bells were going off at every turn. We were no longer able to ignore the signs. Being clumsy and forgetful was one thing, but fighting vertigo and wanting to cry every time I had to face easy tasks such as putting on socks or unloading the dryer was quite another. So I headed to my GP, where I was treated for the vertigo. He gave me a prescription and told me to get more rest. My husband and I have five children between us, ranging in age from seven to twenty-five; we own two separate companies, have two homes in two states, in two time zones, and a dog. Rest was a foreign concept. With the medication, the vertigo cleared up quickly, so I thought I was okay.

Okay lasted about two weeks. The day after Thanksgiving my husband took me shopping in Chicago. We shopped like fools, carrying bags for hours, when suddenly my right hand went numb. We rushed to the car to put the bags away and tried to get my hand to wake up. Big problem: it didn't. In fact it *never* did.

Back in Atlanta the following week I was determined to get some answers. I chose to go back to my GP, but this time I asked a million questions. I was tested for various things and was finally told perhaps I should consider seeing an endocrinologist. By now, of course, it was the peak of the holiday season and most doctors were working short weeks. There were no appointments available. Well I wasn't about to be stopped. Being the creative and assertive person I am, I finally told one of those "Miss sorry-no-appointment-availables" that I would be living in her waiting room until one was. Two days later Dr. Endocrinologist saw me. Of course he was in a hurry and wouldn't listen to me. Sound familiar? He thought I was hypoglycemic and put me to the task of doing the four pricks a day test. For two weeks I was a human pin cushion, but of course the tests came back inconclusive, at which point he told me in his oh-so-sweet way that he didn't think this was a medical issue he could deal with and suggested I go to a neurologist. Of course I just felt crazy. Couldn't anyone tell me what was going on?

The following day I chose to park it at the local neurologist. This time it only took a few hours of "sitting in" for him to see me. He listened intently, tested me extensively, electrodes and all, and encouraged me to have an MRI, which I did.

The following day the doctor himself called from his cell phone to tell me that he thought I had demyelination of the central nervous system. He said he suspected multiple sclerosis. My first reaction was, "Is that the Jerry Lewis disease?" It's not.

Okay, so now I had a name for what might be wrong, but I didn't really know a thing about MS. I figured I had two choices: either ignore the doctor and live with the weird symptoms or read up on MS and find out what I could do about them. You guessed it. I chose the research route. I went to bookstores, searched the Internet, talked to medical professionals, my parents, a service dog trainer for folks with MS, a physical therapist—you name it, I did it. I wanted control. I wanted knowledge. I wanted to make my own choices.

With the help of family and friends, I found out all sorts of interesting things about MS. I discovered that weight training, stretching, and daily exercise would increase my strength, flexibility and muscle memory so I could potentially continue to walk and write even if I was going numb. I learned that I should be resting when I was tired, working and flying less, and lowering the stress in my life.

I learned that hot weather, heated pools, warm baths, and heavy clothing were not going to be my friends. And I discovered the Swank book and its MS diet of almost no saturated fat; no dairy; limited red meat; and a vitamin cocktail with evening primrose oil, acidophilus, and lecithin—all linked to the possibility of helping MS patients.

Now, what was I supposed to do with all this information? Give up my favorite foods? Take seventy pills a day when only eight are Rx? Force myself to go to the gym to work out by myself or with a trainer every stinking day? Wasn't I supposed to be resting more? Hunh? Should I give up being "super mom" and the kind of company president who handles every detail almost to a fault?

You bet. I was determined to be in charge of my life by taking action, even if it meant making difficult choices. My husband called a family meeting and explained my condition, as we understood it, to our girls. Looking at their sweet, concerned faces was one of the hardest things we had to do, but we wanted to make it as unscary for them as possible.

In the weeks to come my husband and children came up with lists of things other people could do for me. They decided they didn't care who cooked dinner, cleaned the house, washed their clothes, or mowed our lawn. They cared that I ate dinner with them, helped them choose which clean clothes to wear, helped them with projects, and played outside with them. They cared that in our very clean house I was still awake to read to them, pray for them, and kiss them goodnight.

Next I had to talk with my coworkers about the changes I would have to make in my work life. For starters, I would now be coming in around 7:15 A.M. and leaving by 3:00 P.M. so I could go to the gym and work out. No more twelve-hour days. I also had to delegate anything that was not critical for me to do personally. Being an overachiever and type A personality, which by the way seem to go hand in hand with MS in some of the research findings, all this delegating and letting go made me feel out of control at first, but then things started to change. I found that I could plan breakfast or dinner meetings, just not both; when traveling I could always find a hotel with a fitness center so I could work out; and I could usually find restaurants that offered healthier "MS" choices. I began to understand that admitting to our limitations isn't being weak or handicapped, it's being honest.

I still take the prescribed oral drugs to help with the symptoms, inject myself with one of the treatments being used to slow the progression of the disease, take the vitamin cocktail, exercise daily, and eat pretty well—most days. I wear inserts when I am walking long distances, wear my braces if my legs seem to be dragging, and carry my cane with me when I am traveling. I feel like I am taking an active role in my physical health. And much of the time I feel alright.

But, I'm convinced that part of my well-being can be attributed to another life-changing choice I made. As my health kept deteriorating, the fact that I was adopted and didn't know my medical history became more and more problematic. Up to that point I had never had any desire to find my biological parents—I have the greatest parents in the world and they chose me, so why would I?—but now it seemed that I might have to.

I knew I was adopted in Cincinnati, Ohio, so I called the adoption agencies listed in the Cincinnati phone book and discovered that I'd been adopted through the Children's Methodist home, which now had a different name. I called and spoke with an intern there, giving her my date of birth and adopted parents' names. I was lucky. Turns out the state of Ohio started sealing adoption records two months after I was born, so I made it just under the wire. Within a few minutes the intern was able to give me my biological mother's name and address as of the time of my birth, along with her background information—her parents' names, siblings' names, ages, and medical history.

From there I contacted the birth records division for the state of Ohio and gave them the information, and they simply pulled my birth certificate and adoption certificate. The whole thing took about five hours. Incredible.

Okay, now what? I knew my birth mother's name, but I didn't want to just storm into someone's life and make a mess. It was the Friday before Memorial Day, so I decided just to hold tight. About four months later I started thinking about contacting my birth mother again. But I really wanted to do it right, so I called the intern and asked her for the phone numbers of groups that makes the probing phone calls for you. As luck would have it the caller reached my biological mom easily, and my mom assured her that it was okay; she had already told everyone in her life about there being a "me" out there somewhere.

So, after all those years I finally met my birth mother. I must admit it was pretty cool to see where my looks come from. At that point I still hadn't been diagnosed definitively, but I was pretty sure I had MS; ironically, her husband (not my biological father) also had MS, so she had facts and pointers for me.

These days I go around speaking to families who are considering adoption or have just adopted. I encourage open adoption, first and foremost for medical reasons. I can't tell you how many times I had to fill out medical forms and felt so embarrassed because I couldn't answer any of the questions about family medical history. People shouldn't have to go through that. That's why I encourage people not to wait until they need the information as I did.

As I speak with parents, I also let them know what it was like for me growing up as an adopted child. I say to them, "Can you imagine looking in the mirror and wondering why you look like you do? Or if you are ever going to have gray hair and when? Or where some special talent came from? I love my parents with all my heart, but knowing where I come from has been pretty awesome.

I encourage those of you faced with MS to have hope. Do something. Don't sit back and wait for this condition to take you. I thank God I took action. By seeking medical history and information, I have been able to get the best medical treatments available and have the privilege of making a difference in the lives of other adopted children. You see, MS can be a good thing.

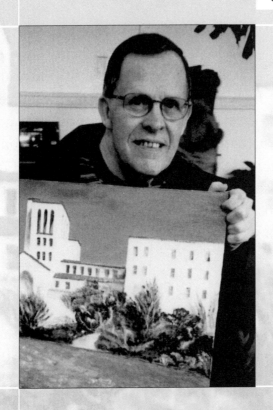

CHAPTER 23

Late Bloomer

BOB NEIL

BECAUSE I HAD SO MUCH SUPPORT here at the hospital, I discovered my love for painting. Since making that discovery, I'm flying high. I've found a kind of healing that cannot be found on any prescription pad but can only come from inside us in a declaration of independence to pursue our creativity. After thirteen years at the hospital, the artist BobbyN. was born. _____

I grew up in a large Catholic family during the Depression. We lived in Spokane, Washington, where I attended Catholic school and church, then moved to San Francisco when I was eleven. We were a close family, and community was always very important. I served in the army after graduating from high school and then attended San Francisco City College's hotel and restaurant program. For several years I worked in the hotel and restaurant industry.

In 1962, I moved to Placerville, California, in the Sierra foothills, to take a job with the California State Automobile Association. That's where I met and married my wife. In 1966 we moved back to San Francisco, where I began a new career in the sporting goods industry, and in 1969 we moved to Petaluma, a farming town about forty-five minutes north of San Francisco. I continued to commute to San Francisco and loved my life. I enjoyed my job, my family, hunting, climbing mountains, fly-fishing, and I spent lots of time outdoors.

But the year 1975 turned my world upside down. I was having trouble walking and standing, my nine-year marriage ended, our fourth child was born without me being present, I lost my job, and I was diagnosed with MS.

Walking out of that doctor's office I felt as if a label had been slapped on my back. It took me two years to peel it off. When I needed family most, I didn't have it, and a deep depression set in. Finally I came to the conclusion that I had three choices: I could jump off the Golden Gate Bridge, pick up drinking, or get my act together. Fortunately I chose the latter.

I moved back to San Francisco, got my own apartment, and went back to college at San Francisco State University. I studied psychology to better understand myself and eventually earned a bachelor's degree in psychology and a master's degree in adult education and counseling.

Knowing I had to be productive, I got involved in the MS Society's Northern California Chapter and did anything I could to help. I stuffed envelopes, became a peer counselor, started a support group, eventually joined the Board of Directors, and spent time fundraising. At the same time I taught ESL (English as a Second Language) to adults in my home. My other volunteer efforts were at Laguna Honda Hospital—a long-term care facility for chronically ill patients. I organized catered lunches for residents with MS.

Over time it became harder and harder to live alone. Driving was becoming difficult as I continued to lose use of my entire right side. I spoke with my doctor, and in 1990 we decided it best for me to move into Laguna Honda Hospital. How ironic. I had visited that place so often but never imagined moving into it myself.

Moving into the hospital was quite a shock, but again, I realized I had choices to make. I could sink into depression in my twelve-by-fifteen-foot room, give up, and let others take care of me and watch me wither away, or I could think of the move as a blessing. I would be relieved of mundane chores such as laundry, meals, and cleaning, and use my time productively. I decided I was still worth something and should enjoy my new freedom.

From my volunteer work at Laguna Honda, I already had friends and knew what services were available. An art instructor at Laguna Honda suggested I try painting. I had no use of my right side, so that would mean going back to "first grade" to learn to write and/or paint with my left hand. This beautiful instructor told me it was entirely possible.

Before long, I discovered a passion and talent for painting. I found that although I was no longer able to hunt and fish, I could now express my love for nature through my paintings of birds, animals, landscapes, and portraits. Now my paintings fill the walls in my room and the corridors at Laguna Honda; my work has been included in an exhibit of art by seniors at the M. H. de Young Memorial Museum; and I've had two other exhibits as well. One of my paintings was chosen to appear in the 2002 National Multiple Sclerosis Society calendar, and just recently, another painting—*Carmine Bee-Eaters,* an acrylic on canvas—was selected for inclusion in the 2003 National Multiple Sclerosis Society calendar.

When I was told that my painting had been selected, they asked me what painting has done for me and what it could do for others. I talked about the elevating clarity of the creative mind and its healing power—a kind of healing that cannot be found on any prescription pad but can only come from inside us in a declaration of independence to pursue our creativity. My hope is that others with MS will see the calendar, all of the artists' work, and become inspired to explore their own creativity in whatever form it may come.

I made myself a promise to remain productive. Here at Laguna Honda, I value our community, just as I did growing up. I chair the Resident Council at Laguna Honda, advocating for residents and reviewing needs and concerns for all 1,100 patients. Although we occasionally have our problems, you would have to travel pretty far to find a facility of this caliber.

My "family" here—residents, volunteers, staff—have helped me battle the degeneration I am experiencing with MS. I encourage residents to get involved in the many activities provided so they too can see the benefits of productivity, creativity, and community involvement.

Society today does not promote the same support systems, the same sense of community I had as a child, but I believe that people simply don't have a chance to develop their lives and their abilities without such community and support. I could have given up when I couldn't live alone, work, or have immediate family take care of me. Instead, I chose long-term care and became blessed with a new family, a new support system.

Because of that support, at sixty-eight I discovered my love for painting. Since making that discovery, I'm flying high. I wish for anyone suffering who believes he or she is alone to take advantage of support systems and rediscover a joyful, fulfilling life.

To view and/or order the 2003 National MS Society calendar: *www.nationalmssociety.org*